DISEASE SIGNS IN THE IRIS

Interpretation and Medication

Theodor Kriege and A. W. Priest

SOCIETY OF IRIDOLOGISTS
80 PORTLAND ROAD
BOURNEMOUTH
BH9 1NQ

L. N. FOWLER & CO. LTD.
1201/3 High Rd., Chadwell Heath
Romford, Essex RM6 4DH

ISBN 0 85243 372 7

Printed and bound in England
by Staples Printers Rochester Limited
at The Stanhope Press

Contents

Part 1

INTERPRETATION AND DIAGNOSIS

Theodor Kriege

Foreword

This book is not intended to be a textbook of irisdiagnosis. In the following work the disease signs are considered and explained as shown in original iris photographs. With few exceptions the conditions have been confirmed by special methods of diagnosis, such as radiographic and blood investigation etc., as well as by subsequent surgical operations.

The disease-signs shown in each illustration of the iris will be explained as they relate to each other and as they must be considered together. This 'considering together' is a basic requirement for iris-diagnosis, since only in this way can the frequently made objection be refuted, that the person whose irides show signs affecting every vital organ consequently must be no longer capable of life. The synthetic approach teaches us that it is never solely a question of only one organ being involved, but that the disturbance in any organ depends upon the total stress affecting all other organs. Therefore, it follows that not merely one organ sign is to be considered, but the causative iris-signs generally form a large and essential part of the assessment. Thus, there is no special sign for tuberculosis or cancer.

Since the irisdiagnostician usually begins by considering the indications of the first major zone, immediately around the pupil (gastro-intestinal zone), I will similarly commence by explaining the signs in this zone. In this connection, the pupil itself and the pupillary margin (so-called 'neurasthenic ring') should not be disregarded. However, since many of the changes affecting the pupillary margin are not clearly recognisable from the illustrations, I will include in my discussion only those which can be seen perfectly.

Notes extracted from the clinical case records are appended to the descriptions of the individual iris illustrations.

After studying the illustrations, the reader may come to a

different interpretation or significance concerning the various signs. Apart from the fact that my diagnosis has been made on the basis of forty years practical experience, the reader should also remember that other methods of examination may provide the basis for different interpretations of the same disease syndrome, as may be possible, for example, with radiographic diagnosis. Herewith an example: A patient, B.H. from O, a large, powerful and well-nourished man, consulted me. He complained of neuralgic pains affecting variable locations and which were very troublesome. According to his statement the complaint had existed for several years. After taking the case-history, I proceeded to examination. All the usual clinical investigations gave no clear picture, whereas the examination of the iris clearly showed a focal infection of the teeth, to which the neuralgic pains were due. The patient then explained to me that he had suffered toothache frequently, and although the dentist had wished to radiograph the teeth, he had not yet done so.

On further examination, the patient asked me whether his stomach was healthy. I had said nothing about it. I then explained that because of faulty nutrition in youth a condition of gastro-intestinal catarrh had developed and still persisted. From an earlier state of chronic ulceration, scar tissue and adhesions affected much of the stomach, which gave rise to recurrent complaint. To his question as to whether an operation would eventually become necessary, I replied that such an operation would be bad, since the condition would require the removal of the whole stomach. On hearing this the patient expressed his pleasure to find confirmed that which a professor in Cologne had told him five years before, namely that his stomach was one great continuous cicatrisation, and that it was not possible to operate. Another radiologist could not find any significant change in the stomach in spite of repeated examination by radiography. How it arises that two such different diagnoses can be made, I cannot judge. For the practitioner it should be a warning not to regard his diagnosis as wrong before the contrary has been completely demonstrated.

The photographs shown in this book date from 1938. Following the topographical iris-chart of Frau Eva Flink, I have used the basic division of the iris into three major zones (= six minor zones), and in order to achieve standardisation of terms, the six minor zones are designated as follows—

1st minor zone—stomach zone.	4th minor zone—muscle zone.
2nd minor zone—intestinal zone.	5th minor zone—bone zone.
3rd minor zone—blood zone.	6th minor zone—mucous membrane and skin zone.

Reference to the position of individual organs is indicated by the word 'area' e.g. kidney area, heart area, etc.

For easier location of the various signs and indications I have chosen to divide the iris circle into 'minutes' i.e. 1-60 minutes in each iris, using the usual apostrophe (') to avoid confusion.

The older designation—'loss-of-substance sign' is here replaced by the term—'defect sign'.

Understanding the following material requires a knowledge of the basic concepts as presented in my textbook "Fundamental Basis of Irisdiagnosis—a concise textbook".

The suggestion for the first edition of the following work was made to me by my teacher, Frau Eva Flink, to whom I wish to express my indebtedness and gratitude.

Osnabrück 1969   Theodor Kriege

Introduction

Following the usual practice in irisdiagnosis, we begin with a consideration of the stomach ring.

The cardia lies to the left of the midline of the trunk and is located therefore in the upper half of the left iris, at 45-50′ and 10-15′ in the first minor zone. In my view, the position of the cardia should not be placed in the lower half of the iris. The pylorus, which lies to the right of the midline, is similarly located at 12-18′ and 42-48′ in the first minor zone of the right iris.

Anatomically, the duodenum is subdivided into an upper, a vertical, a horizontal and a descending section, (Pars superior, Pars ascendens, Pars horizontales and Pars descendens), the signs for which at 38-45′ in the right iris extend outward into the second minor zone. Like the pylorus, the duodenum as far as the Pars ascendens lies on the right side of the body, so that the signs for these parts are to be located in the right iris as follows—

Pylorus generally—at 15′.

Terminal pylorus and commencement of the duodenum at 40-45′ in the first minor zone (stomach zone).

Duodenum as far as the horizontal section at 38-48′ in the second minor zone (intestinal zone).

Signs for the horizontal section of the duodenum are to be located in the second minor zone (intestinal zone) at 20-25′, and the last part: ascending section including the flexure to the small intestine, at 38-40′ in the second minor zone of the left iris.

In order the better to understand those iris signs which appear when there are duodenal disturbances, the connection of the duodenum with other organs should be reviewed—

The posterior wall of the stomach is in contact with the spleen, the left kidney and suprarenal gland, and the pancreas. The lesser curvature of the stomach is covered by the left lobe of the liver, and the greater curvature is adjacent to the transverse colon.

The beginning of the duodenum, the common bile duct and the pancreas, are in close proximity; the descending part of the duodenum is adjacent to the right kidney, transverse colon and pancreas, while the horizontal section contacts the pancreas. The last part of the duodenum (ascending) is likewise contiguous with the pancreas and has its flexure very close to the stomach.

The great blood vessels—abdominal aorta and lower vena cava, together with the omental vessels—lie in the immediate neighbourhood of the duodenum.

If these facts are considered, it will be evident that when disease processes affect the pylorus, duodenum or pancreas, then neighbouring structures can be disturbed. To demonstrate: where inflammatory adhesions affect the descending part of the duodenum, then the pancreas, kidney and colon may be affected by adhesions, resulting in disturbances which may vary according to circumstances, the extent of the adhesions and the side affected. Similarly, obstruction of the bile and pancreatic duct at its orifice will induce stasis in the organs: liver, gall-bladder and pancreas.

All these disturbances are portrayed in the iris. The signs are to be seen not only in the intestinal zone (L.38-40′), but also, when the pancreas is involved, in the third and fourth minor zones in the areas for pancreas. The signs are appropriate to the kind of disturbance: if the kidney is involved, then a kidney sign will be found; if the local condition affects the blood vessels, such as the portal vein or the gastric or hepatic vessels, then signs will be found in the blood zone.

Taking these various relations into consideration, the signs in the different organ areas and zones will be fully explained when they stand in connection with the causative conditions.

The typical difference of the signs for particular locations should also be noted. Ulcerative states affecting the stomach are shown by black spots in the first minor zone, whereas ulcerations affecting the pylorus and duodenum are seldom found as black spots, but rather more elongated black signs. The basis for this difference is not yet clear.

At the beginning of any disease process just a small white sign is to be seen (white cloud = inflammation sign). Should the inflammation involve neighbouring organs, then adhesions will appear in the same way as happens with inflammation of the pleura. If the inflammation is without suppuration, then only small white, oblique lines are to be seen (transversals = adhesion signs) as the reaction declines. Where however the process is suppurative and tissue loss is already apparent, then the iris will show one or more black signs in association with the adhesion signs (defect signs = loss-of-substance signs).

If during the course of illness adhesions develop which restrict the function of contiguous organs, then appropriate signs will appear in the affected organ areas. These signs may indicate displacement of the border of stomach and intestinal zones, dark lacunae to show weakness, and dark to black signs in all forms to indicate dense scar tissue.

The evidence of iris findings suggests that most disturbances arise through absorption of foreign material from the digestive organs (intestinal intoxication) and insufficient elimination of these toxic substances and destructive metabolic residues through the kidneys, bowel and skin. That severe disturbances can arise through dysbacteria and auto-intoxication has been known for a long time.

If the processing organs of the first major zone are diseased, foreign materials are conveyed from these organs to those of the second major zone, ultimately resulting in their failure, as also of the kidneys and skin, the principal eliminative organs. It is the normal function of these organs to eliminate destructive metabolic wastes.

The lymphatic system, which extends throughout the organism and stands in close connection with the blood vascular system, merits greater attention than it has so far received, bearing in mind that the lacteals of the intestinal villi are the origin of the gastro-intestinal lymph system, and are responsible for taking up those toxic materials from the gut which provide the basis for diseases in the whole body. Signs proclaiming disease affecting the lymphatic system (lymphatic constitution) are to be found extending outwards from the autonomic wreath, i.e. in the ciliary zone (second and third major zones).

The assertion that most diseases probably originate from the stomach and intestines may now be explained in somewhat greater detail. The principal nutrients are protein, fat and carbohydrate. A disturbance will appear consequent upon over or under-nourishment with any one of these nutrients and give rise to the development of a corresponding sign in the iris.

Over- or undernourishment with any one of the principal nutrients, protein, fat or carbohydrate, will result in a corresponding disturbance and show an appropriate sign in the iris. This phenomenon is most easily seen in the eyes of small children, where even as early as one month after birth the stomach and intestinal zones show intensely white colouring. When these signs appear, one may certainly conclude that there is over-feeding of carbohydrate in the form of sugar and white flour products. The children at first appear well nourished but possess little energy and are quiet.

With deterioration of the condition, white peaks develop proceeding outwards from the iris-wreath, eventually connecting by radiating white lines with small to large white clouds located in the third major zone (so-called "lymph-bridges"), dark spots appear in the intestinal area, kidney signs appear, and a dark to black scurf rim develops in the sixth minor zone. Similar signs are also found in the intestinal ring and lymph system where there has been over-consumption of fats, but the signs are less snow-white in intensity and tend somewhat towards yellow.

A disturbance arising from protein over-consumption is seldom in question with children, since a high protein intake is required for growth. However, protein can be dangerous in the presence of a diseased or ulcerated state of the gastro-intestinal mucosa (recognised by black spots in the iris areas), since there may be absorption of toxic material in the form of insufficiently reduced foreign protein which seriously encumbers the lymphatic system. In this situation, small dark spots appear in the second and third major zones (ciliary area), signifying that the lymph nodes have declined in their capacity of resistance and now serve as foci of precipitated toxic material. Further deterioration by way of purulent decomposition is the next possibility.

If on this background infectious disease or other toxic conditions arise which overcome local resistance and affect the whole nervous system, then signs of varied colours appear in all areas of the iris. The lack of vitamins may also produce severe disturbances, but generally there is also a perverted or unbalanced nutrition.

It should be noted especially that in the case of excessive intake

14

of refined carbohydrates in the form of white flour and white sugar products, a calcium deficiency condition will arise which cannot be remedied simply by supplying increased vitamin D, since in the absence of sufficient calcium and phosphorus the vitamin D is unable to influence the condition. In this context vitamin C is also required for calcium transportation. In the presence of constitutional damage from calcium deficiency the well-known nerve rings are seen in the iris.

If as a result of all these conditions the glandular organs such as the liver, pancreas, suprarenal glands, pituitary, thyroid and parathyroid glands suffer permanent damage, then severe chronic diseases such as diabetes, Addison's disease, etc., may develop and dark signs will appear in the appropriate organ areas of the iris.

That not all such chronic diseases will develop in every patient is clear, for hereditary tendency will in the one case favour this, and in the other case that form of disease. In this matter the particular constitution with its predisposition provides a certain diagnostic possibility and which, on the appearance of the first signs of disturbance, enables one to predict the probable consequences if an energetic correction of faulty nutrition is not made.

Iris-1 has been chosen to demonstrate the ring zones, especially the third to sixth minor zones. The first minor zone is seen as a large, grey circle, immediately around the pupil, which is itself somewhat enlarged. The second minor zone extends from the grey stomach ring to the iris-wreath (shown by the intensely white, indented circle). The intestinal ring, however, is only visible as such between 60' to 30' and 38' to 55'.

The outer demarcation of the second major zone is never so positively indicated as the outer limit of the first major zone, which as the iris-wreath is almost always visible. If the area lying outside the iris-wreath (ciliary area) is divided into two equally wide circles, then it is seen that the inner circle is more coarsely textured than the outer, showing alternating open and closed lacunae (= dark oval signs).

Subdividing the middle circle (second major zone) into two rings of equal width produces the third minor zone (blood and lymph) and the fourth minor zone (muscle). Within these two zones are found the signs for conditions affecting blood and muscle tissue in general, as well as the organs projected in these zones: heart, kidneys, suprarenal glands, pancreas and pituitary gland.

The third major zone, extending from the outer limit of the muscle zone to the iris-margin, is also subdivided into two circles: the fifth minor zone (bone) and the sixth minor zone (mucous membrane/skin). The brain and the sexual organs are projected in these two zones.

However, as in the organism so in the iris, there is no rigid demarcation. Everything is mobile. Thus, in general deficiency of the blood (anaemia) it is found that according to the severity of the condition the effects (lacunae) extend over the iris zones, reaching to the iris margin, as seen in Iris-1 at 52-54' and 47-49'. These lacunae are to be distinguished from defect-signs (tissue damage) which can be observed as black signs enclosed by a white border at 30' in the area for the leg. (A closed lacuna is seen at 27', adjacent to these defect-signs).

In presenting Iris-1 as an ideal iris, it is not to be assumed that this iris shows no signs of disease. On the contrary, there are many.

17

But a patient showing such an iris will quickly recover from any acute condition on account of the healthy skin function, which leaves the organism less encumbered in spite of reduced renal activity. This last condition is to be seen from the dark sign at 31' in the second major zone which includes a long black sign.

Turning the attention to Iris-2, one is immediately impressed by the poor skin function, indicated by the wide and almost black skin zone. The poor surface elimination has resulted in the accumulation of much metabolic waste within the organism. The kidney area (30-38') is particularly encumbered. As principal eliminative organs, the kidneys cannot carry this burden and ultimately fail. If in such a condition no value is to be accorded to elimination by the skin and kidneys, then no improvement can be expected in any disease condition.

The difference in external appearance between these two patients is:

Patient Iris-1: slender, lean person with nervous weakness and ready perspiration.

Patient Iris-2: small and corpulent, bloated person with a puffy, pallid and yellow appearance. Lack of perspiration.

Treatment of the skin with oil would be useful for both patients. The first requires peaceful surroundings and no exertions, whereas the second needs treatment by hot and sauna baths, packs, and physical activity to the point of active perspiration.

Both patients have a lymphatic constitution. There is in both a tendency to skin conditions originating in disorder of the lymphatic system. (Faulty nutrition, thereby disturbance of stomach and intestines). In Iris-1, weakness of the blood and nervous system shows prominently, and because of nervous exhaustion, perspiration is too profuse. Quite the opposite is the case with Iris-2. Here, the very poor circulation to the skin is due to marked over-contraction of the capillaries, resulting in congestive inflammation of the organs and leading to disturbances which are quite different from those presented in Iris-1.

In the former case (Iris-1), nerve pains may appear, whereas in the latter case muscular pains are probable. From the internal congestion and toxic influences affecting the stomach and intestine shown in Iris-2, there arises the exessively light colouring of the gastro-intestinal zone. The small first major zone (note the iris-wreath) shows over-stimulation of the vegetative nervous system, while the black streaks radiating from the pupillary margin result from central nervous exhaustion.

Although Iris-1 shows that toxic material from the intestinal disturbance is absorbed into the blood and lymph stream, indicated by the excessively white colouring of the iris-wreath and the light radiations into the second major zone, yet there is good elimination of the material through the skin (heavy perspiration), as shown by the skin zone.

It is otherwise with Iris-2. In this case, the tendency to inflammatory reaction of the inner organs, as shown by the strong white colouring of the fifth minor zone, arises from the complete cessation of skin function. However, it is not only the skin condition which is to blame for the disturbances suffered by this patient, but also the renal failure.

Commencing at 30', at the narrowed intestinal zone, Iris-1 shows a healed lesion of the kidney, the result of inflammation and tissue damage. This is indicated by the three small, long, black signs within the kidney sign. (A)

Iris-2 shows a sign at 26' to 34', originating at the pupillary margin and extending outwards and widthwise as far as the sixth minor zone. This sign is so wide in the sixth zone that the area between the two white arcs at 26' and 35' should be regarded as one sign. This large sign, showing an intensely white surrounding border, indicates that the function of the left kidney has suffered extensively (renal stasis). Nevertheless, there may be no evidence of any disease in the urine. The significance of the spleen sign will be discussed later. (B)

The encumbrance of the spleen shown in Iris-2 is seen not only from the particularly dark colouring of the third major zone between 17' and 25', but also from the displacement of the white signs towards the pupil in the same segment. Swelling of the spleen is shown by the widening of the dark scurf rim with flattening of the peripheral border. Febrile reactions are always to be expected with such a large spleen. (C)

In Iris-1 there is a large gastro-intestinal zone (first major zone), the iris-wreath enclosing about one-third of the iris, which is considered normal. In Iris-2 the iris-wreath is contracted inwards and almost to the pupil. This shows the difference of nervous stress. In Iris-1 a weakness of the vegetative nervous system is indicated, although the function of the central nervous system is well sustained. In Iris-2, there is an over-sensitivity of the vegetative nervous system and the central nervous system is weakened. This explains the basic difference between the two patients as described above.

The patient with Iris-1 has a tendency to neurosis. In my experience, such patients are especially prone to develop infantile paralysis during the years of childhood. The patient with Iris-2 tends to suffer severe anaemia and rheumatic muscular pains.

At 15′, in the second major zone of Iris-1, there is a not very clearly demarcated dark sign, suggestive of a damaged heart valve. There are several quite small black points also to be seen in the heart area between 11′ and 17′. These small points indicate myocardial damage. In this case they are only quite small foci in the heart muscle and probably not clinically verifiable. The two white lines which extend from the pupillary margin to the iris rim indicate over-stimulation of the nerve supply to the heart and suggest the possibility of cardiac neurosis. (D)

At 15′ in the third minor zone of Iris-2 there is also a small narrow black defect-sign which can be regarded as a healed lesion. It is difficult to see whether a black point is to be found at this sign which would signify a valvular lesion. Immediately below the sign, two sharply defined white lines extend almost as far as the iris-rim, suggesting a state of cardiac neurosis. (E)

Referring to Iris-1, consider the large lacuna at 27-29′, which begins in a contracted part of the iris-wreath and extends as far as the sixth minor zone. This indicates weakness and disturbance of the suprarenal function, and being in the left iris has a special significance: dysfunction of the vegetative nervous system with a tendency to emaciation, disturbances of the circulation with cardiac and gastro-intestinal symptoms. Close observation shows the sign to be somewhat obliquely inclined from 29′ at the iris-wreath to the outer iris-rim, suggesting possible displacement. (F)

The interrupted thin black line, which begins at 26′ in an indentation of the wreath line and extends to meet the iris-rim at 25′, also shows displacement. Displacements are also indicated by the oblique arclines which begin at 22′ and 20′ in the second major zone to terminate at 25′ and 23′ respectively in the third major zone. In addition, there is a slight displacement of the wreath line upwards in the section from 20′ to 30′, which would otherwise be expected to show a dilatation. All these signs are suggestive of displacement within the abdominal cavity, which arise not only from the kidney and suprarenal conditions but possibly from cystic development having its origin in the right ovary. In view of these signs, confirmatory evidence should be sought in the areas for uterus and ovary in the right iris. (G)

To the signs for displacement in the abdominal cavity shown between 20′ and 30′ are to be added those oblique white arc lines seen at 36-38′ covering the area for rectum and bladder as far as the back.

The signs for haemorrhoids are not only the thick white lines which extend from the iris-wreath to the iris-margin at 35′, but also the black pointed sign inside the wreath at 36′, as well as the dark signs at 24′ in the second minor zone. These last signs indicate mucous membrane catarrh and erosions affecting the sigmoid colon, producing a continuous rectal discharge and consequent burning, irritation and soreness of the anus. (H)

The sign at 38′ in the area for bladder, including the intensely white cloud adjacent to the iris-wreath, suggests burning on micturition. The extension of the white line to the iris-rim indicates vaginal and vulval irritation. The symptoms present with such signs are almost never reported by the patient but are confirmed on interrogation. Moreover, the presence of abdominal cysts can exist for many years without giving rise to symptoms, or the symptoms are attributed to gastro-intestinal disturbances. (J)

Considering now the group of signs in the fifth minor zone between 38′ and 44′ in the area for the back, together with the arclines adjacent to the iris-wreath between 6′ and 12′, suggests that adjustment of the cervical vertebrae could have a beneficial influence upon the whole condition.

Referring to the large dark sign in the spleen sector of Iris-2, at 18-25′ in the second and third major zones, it is evident that apart from enlargement there is also some tissue damage, as shown by the small black sign at 25′ within the darkened area. The transversal which half encloses this sign, turns inwards and upwards at 20′ to the heart area. (C) In these cases there may be frequent cardiac spasms, which have nothing to do with the coronary vessels but probably arise from digestive conditions. It is often found with such patients that the most severe condition affects the pancreas, producing digestive disturbance from obstruction of the pancreatic duct. This gives rise to flatulence and consequent pressure upon the diaphragm, leading to the gastro-cardiac syndrome. In relation to this, consider the long black sign at 22′ adjacent to the iris-wreath in the second major zone. It is to be regarded as a pancreas sign and indicates tissue damage affecting the tail of the pancreas. This raises the question of diabetes, although there may be no evident glycosuria. (K)

The small, long black sign, beginning at the iris-wreath at 30′ and ending at 26′ in the fourth minor zone, is a suprarenal sign which is displaced towards 25′, this confirming the kidney disease described above. Note the white line beginning at the iris-rim at 37′ and running across obliquely to 40′ in the second major zone, from which point it again runs out to the iris-rim, thus forming an angle. This sign suggests that some influence from outside has affected the lumbar vertebrae and the sacrum. Taken together with the sign complex at 5-10′ in the second and third major zones, adjustment of vertebrae in the neck and back should be considered. (L)

These signs probably refer to a spinal injury as being the cause of the kidney condition (floating kidney), as well as of the conditions affecting the suprarenal gland, pancreas (tissue damage and displacement), spleen (tissue damage and enlargement) and even the diaphragm and the heart. The patient's statement indicates that none of the many treatments given took these connections into account. The true state of affairs was revealed only after careful consideration of the iris photographs.

Case record of Patient—1:
Housewife, 32 years of age, married with one child. History of one miscarriage.
Father 65 years old, mother 59 years old and suffers from anaemia. Of the four brothers and sisters of the father, two died from heart failure and one sister from tuberculosis.
Previous illnesses: measles with renal complications, mumps, influenza. On the birth of the child by forceps delivery a small laceration was suffered and the patient developed eclampsia. The child who is now nine years of age also shows an oblique line in the iris, especially on the left side.
The symptoms recorded at the first consultation were: red, painless flecks on the right leg which had been there for two years, otherwise suffers haemorrhoids and occasional headaches.

Case record of Patient—2:

Housewife, 31 years of age, the fourth child of five children. (One sister died of heart failure at 19 years of age.) Married with no children.

The father suffers from a heart condition. The mother is healthy. One sister of the mother died from tuberculosis at the age of 23 years. Both maternal grandparents died from influenza at the ages of 46 years and 56 years respectively.

The symptoms recorded at the first consultation were: asthmatic attacks and susceptibility to colds; rough, irritable and easily inflamed skin; adhesions affecting the pleura and ovaries.

The asthmatic attacks and the susceptibility to colds were improved after a short time. The following statement was made by the patient herself—

"I had measles when I was a small child. At twelve years of age I went down with six days of influenza and ten days of measles, following which I had frequent cardiac palpitations and headaches and the skin sensitivity appeared. The doctor called the skin reaction—dermographia, found it very interesting but otherwise without significance. At that time it was established that the heart was too small, but nothing was done. In 1930 I collapsed from total physical exhaustion and for about six months my temperature was raised. For the second time I was told that I probably imagined my complaint. In 1932 I was operated upon for appendicitis and had not yet recovered when my brother had to undertake a very severe operation. For fourteen days I was awake both day and night. Later I lay in hospital for three weeks because of considerable pains from the operation scars and recovered only with difficulty. I suffered frequently from breathlessness and heart symptoms. In 1934 I was for nine months under treatment with a heilpraktiker, who established that I had suffered from asthma for a long time and was otherwise not healthy. I was treated with injections but the condition progressively worsened. In the winter of 1938 I suffered glandular inflammation for six weeks and in the mid-summer of 1939 I had pleurisy for four weeks. Since that time I have been particularly susceptible. In the spring of 1940 I undertook a cure in Bad Sooden-Allendorf. The spa doctor told me that my little cough was nothing to worry about and my heart was amazingly healthy. After fourteen days treatment he was of a different opinion. Now I am extraordinarily sensitive and since the autumn of 1939 I have already had a severe cold three times."

In this iris photograph the stomach zone (first minor zone) is not very clearly defined. However, it is still easily distinguished from the intestinal zone (second minor zone) and the outer border of the stomach zone is easily recognised.

The light coloured stomach area, with its small black spokes radiating from the pupillary margin, is the expression of an inflammatory over-stimulation of the stomach muscle layer, which leads to a coarseness of the gastric mucosal convolutions and to degeneration of the mucosa. These signs generally arise from a disturbed blood circulation resulting from neurogenic spasm, with the consequence that the gastric mucous membrane is no longer adequately nourished and therefore loses its functional efficiency.

A patient showing this stomach ring will not necessarily come to the consulting room complaining of a stomach condition, and should not be described as having a gastric disease. In such a case the disturbance will lie in the arterial vascular system, whereby stasis of the blood circulation takes place in the muscle layer of the stomach, the gastric mucous membrane is less supplied with blood and tends towards atrophy (dark signs without inflammation signs). Therefore stomach symptoms only occur from time to time.

The intestinal zone (second minor zone) is easily seen. It extends from the outer border of the stomach zone to the white iris-wreath. Indications of disease conditions are to be seen in the large, long dark signs at 4′, 10′, 15-20′, 33′, 37′, 44′, 50′ and 54′, as well as in the brilliant white colouring of the iris-wreath. The dark signs are referred to as lacunae (weakness signs) and suggest conditions of debility or over-relaxation of the intestinal musculature.

White lines represent an inflammatory stimulation or irritation of the intestinal mucous membrane. This mucosal inflammation has its origin in an intestinal catarrh of infancy, as shown by the round outward dilatations of the border (wreath). As the result of chronic irritation, such as the long term influence of faulty nutrition, chill and intestinal worms, the catarrh was not resolved. Typical worm signs are to be seen at 5′, 33′, 35′, 50′ and 54′. The case history shows frequent attacks of diarrhoea without pain, and during childhood much diarrhoea and intestinal worms.

Within the heart area (10-15′—third and fourth minor zones), two small closed lacunae are to be seen forming part of the iris-wreath. The smaller, almost point-like sign is to be considered as a defect-sign. These signs have probably formed during childhood, since the patient contracted many severe childhood diseases (A). The large closed lacuna with a white sign immediately below, signifies that there has been a condition of the pericardium involving adhesions to the diaphragm (B).

The lacunae lying obliquely one under the other which are not closed, indicate myocardial weakness and enlargement. This would be significant in acute febrile reactions since cardiac paralysis can easily follow. The white lines radiating from the pupillary margin, together with the inward displacement of the iris-wreath, show that there is a disturbance of the vegetative nervous system with sudden attacks of palpitation (C).

Now observe the small closed lacuna at 28′ in the second major zone. It indicates an old suprarenal lesion which occurred early in youth, implicating the nervous system in such a way as to produce life-long over-stimulation (D). Diametrically opposite, at 57′ in the second and third major zones, a heavy darkened area surrounded by a light cloud-like border is seen. This shows an old, but still active, disturbance of the pituitary body (E).

At 27-28′, in the third major zone, a darkened area with a large white cloud and a small white flake indicate chronic inflammation of the left ovary (F). There is also a dark sign to be seen in the uterus area of the right iris. The association of all these signs explains why the physical and emotional state of the patient is so bad that it costs her much effort to exercise general control. If these sign relations are correctly understood, then it is possible to inform the patient of the ways in which she suffers without having to wait to ask her for details.

To summarise the basic indications: the iris structure is fine and compact, implying an excessively sensitive organism. The conditions affecting stomach and intestines allow no healthy development and prevent adequate recovery after acute phases of organs represented in the ciliary zones. The second major zone is on the whole dark, suggesting a general weakness (anaemia). The heart signs indicate restlessness and anxiety with palpitations. The suprarenal signs indicate vegetative dystony, with disturbances involving the entire blood and lymph circulation and the endocrine system. The pituitary sign shows the influence affecting endocrine (procreative) function, while the ovary/uterus signs implicate the mento-emotional life.

Some further details of the case history may now be added: After five years of marriage the patient gave birth to her first child. The child was never well, had protruding ears with mis-shaped jaw and teeth, thick development of the back of the head, a thick abdomen and thin arms and legs. It died at the age of seventeen years from diphtheria. Five years after the first childbirth, the patient suffered a miscarriage. Her menstruation was always irregular and heavy.

The many large and small white clouds in the third major zone are in general the expression of chronic over-stimulation involving the serous membranes and secondary to the over-burdened lymphatic system. These signs always appear in the upper (= anterior) iris layer and are joined by thick white lines with the iris-wreath ('lymph-bridges'). They are clearly seen in the section 10-20′, where they are particularly large, indicating the heaviest encumbrance and showing the greatest potential for inflammatory reaction. This applies particularly to the regions for shoulder, chest and arm. The white flakes between 40′ and 45′ indicate encumbrance of the back, while those between 45′ and 50′ refer to the mouth and throat as far as the naso-pharynx.

Similar signs between 20′ and 30′ indicate that the abdominal region is affected, as also the areas for leg (30′) and rectum (35′). The patient will confirm a chronic susceptibility to colds, coughs and catarrh of the throat, and of repeated attacks of pain in shoulder and arm, with prominent heart symptoms. All these symptoms are worse in the mornings and aggravated by gales and thunderstorms.

The long weakness sign at 35′, which commences at the iris-wreath and extends outwards to the iris-rim, indicates atony of the anus and ampulla. The narrowed middle section of the sign suggests that the rectum is being compressed by another organ (uterus). In this connection, note the almost round sign at 37′ in the third major zone. This is the cause of the anal condition, since it must refer to enlargement and displacement of the uterus, so that even a soft stool can only be passed with difficulty. Confirmation of the condition should be sought in the uterus area of the right iris. (G)

The large, dark signs appearing in the segment 40-50′ in the second major zone are especially striking. The dark signs between 40′ and 45′ in the third major zone, with the associated white clouds, are in the pleural area of the back. Together with the fine white cross lines, these signs suggest that an old condition of pleurisy has produced adhesions. The fine white oblique and cross lines in the area 15-20′ in the third major zone indicate that the anterior internal surface of the thorax has also participated in the inflammatory reaction with the production of adhesions. In similar cases, the diagnosis will always be confirmed by thoracic radiography. However, what cannot be radiographically ascertained is the state of potential inflammatory reaction of the affected tissues, including the mucous membranes, and of the lymphatic system, to be recognised by the white clouds.

Turning to the signs between 45′ and 50′ and referring to the area for throat, mouth and nose, whenever there have been pulmonary disturbances which have not fully resolved, then the mucous membranes of these organs participate in the residual condition. The large open lacuna at 45′, commencing at the iris-wreath, shows encumbrance of the tonsils, larynx and thyroid gland (H). Where the iris-wreath deviates towards the pupil it suggests that there was a severe inflammatory reaction and that the contiguous organs, such as the oesophagus, were implicated. The deviations of the wreath-line are always to be regarded as indicating disturbance of the vegetative nervous system.

In view of the poor definition of the upper quadrant of the photograph, interpretation of the signs in these areas is not possible.

Iris—4   **Male: 28 years—left iris**

In this picture the outer border of the stomach is not very clearly defined, and there is no striking difference of colour in comparison with the rest of the iris. Therefore, no important pathological activity is evident in relation to the gastro-intestinal system.

The black stain appearing at 48-50′ is in reality of a brown colour, and is not a sign for a stomach condition but indicates a toxin deposit. The edge of the pupil cannot be clearly identified from the picture and might not be very distinct even in the living subject. It would be better indicated by colour photography.

On considering the pupillary margin more closely, three small indentations will be found at 52′, 55′ and 60′, which refer to the nervous system, i.e. the brain (see Schnabel: deformation of the pupil). Also note the dark rhombus-shaped sign at 37′ which commences at the pupil and traverses the bladder area as far as the outer border of the iris (Ear-bladder line) and which includes a small black rhombus-like sign at the intestinal border. This sign is not to be regarded as indicating a gastro-intestinal condition, but should be interpreted together with the toxin deposit and the three small indentations of the pupillary margin.

The white arc-lines (transversals) which commence at the iris-wreath at 13′ and extend downwards to meet the iris-rim at 17′ indicate disturbance of the coronary vessels. The half-moon shaped black sign at 10′ in the third minor zone also indicates enlargement of the aorta (A). These signs are to be interpreted in association with the long black sign in the bladder area which extends to the iris-rim at 38′ (B), the sign for the suprarenal body (30) and the sign for pituitary body (58-59′). Also note the kidney and suprarenal signs.

The expansion of the thick white double lines at 35′, which encloses a small black sign (= defect-sign), suggests that there has been a chronic weakness of the rectum with suppurative conditions (C). That the symptoms are no longer very severe, may be deduced from the absence of white zig-zag lines or white flakes in the area. However, the dark wisp signs which proceed from the outer black point to the iris-rim show that the condition has not yet resolved.

The small dark to black points which are distributed over the whole of the sixth minor zone (skin zone) are signs for ulcers, both existing and potential.

The sign at 38′ has already been referred to in relation to the small localised indentations of the pupillary margin (Ear-bladder line). The half-moon shaped black sign at 10′, the three small black signs at 5′ in the third minor zone, the suprarenal sign at 30′ and the pituitary sign at 58′-59′ have all been mentioned and can now be explained in terms of the total condition.

When signs are to be seen in the bladder area of the left iris (B), they are an indication to the practitioner that systemic conditions are arising from infection, including venereal infection. How are these signs to be interpreted? Since the sign begins at the pupillary margin, thus relating to the central nervous system, and then displaces and breaks through the iris-wreath, it is to be assumed that there is an inner cause. (In the case of outside causes, the wreath is displaced towards the pupil). Because of mental and perhaps emotional defects (hereditary tendency), it is probable that the patient is inclined to sexual over-stimulation. Consequently, restrictions are ignored and precautionary measures disregarded. The result is infection, which encroaches upon the system and destroys weakened organs.

The large dark area in the cerebral region, lying opposite the white uro-genital area, suggests that the increased blood supply to the pelvic organs results in a diminished supply to the head. This indication is also found in younger patients who masturbate. The disturbance of the gonads ultimately affects the pituitary gland and the suprarenal body, which in turn affect the vegetative nervous system, to produce over-contraction of the vascular system and special pathology of the heart and aorta. If there is no control of the excessive indulgence, there develops a condition of emotional depression and ultimately mental degeneration. If, however, the sexual activities are terminated by the development of infection, the iris signs will show the effects of toxaemia in such conditions as rheumatism, gastric crises and cerebral softening, which are difficult to relieve.

In my experience, such conditions are not solely due to hereditary disposition, but are greatly influenced by nourishment and development in youth. I have found in several cases that the excessive ingestion of raw eggs has induced increased sexual activity in young persons, and also that the excessive consumption of seed-germ or seed-germ oil can lead to severe consequences. In gonadal deficiency conditions these substances are able to bring an improvement, if the sexual life is properly conducted.

To return to the iris signs. The long black sign at 38' (B) shows catarrh of the urethra and bladder, and since the sign extends as far as the pupillary margin, it suggests involvement of the vegetative and central nervous systems. The small black signs lying opposite at 5', adjacent to the iris-wreath, indicate disturbance of the carotid artery (hardening, contracture). Two arc lines are seen to be enclosing one of the small black signs which then disappear as they extend towards the iris-rim (D). These lines show the early development of a lacuna and indicate weakening of the tissues.

If, as here, signs are seen which extend towards the outer iris-rim in this area, there will be some developmental difficulty affecting the sense of hearing. A similar disturbance of hearing can also appear when the antecedents of the patient suffered from a disease of the generative organs. (Forefathers-bladder-conditions = Children-ear-conditions).

The half-moon shaped dark to black sign at 10′ indicates aortic enlargement (aneurysm), which has developed with the premature coronary sclerosis (A). The large sign in the area for the pituitary (E) lies opposite the suprarenal sign (F). Since both signs are not yet closed, the conditions may still be influenced. However, the pituitary sign is very large and is contiguous with the dark signs in the upper part of the brain area, indicating that the pituitary disturbance is the cause of the suprarenal condition.

Now consider the large dark open lacuna which commences within the peak at 54′ and extends to the iris-rim (G). This area represents the frontal sinus and raises the question of a possible condition of ozoena. Those with clinical experience of this problem will be aware of the possible causes and the difficulties of treatment.

The thick white deposits surrounding the last two signs described, indicate increased lymphatic activity. This detoxicating activity utilises the mucous membranes of the frontal and maxillary sinuses to produce mucous discharges. Should the patient complain of periodic stomach pains which prove to be resistant to the usual treatment, it may be assumed that these symptoms result from gastric crises.

The case card reads as follows: At the first consultation the patient complained of urethral discharge and was referred immediately to a specialist.

Iris-5   **Male: 24 years—left iris**

In comparison with the previous picture, the stomach zone of this iris is more intensely white and also more sharply defined. Increased whiteness is the sign for gastric hyper-acidity, while the sharper demarcation indicates the tendency to stomach cramp. It could be said of this patient that he suffers from a sense of pressure in the stomach together with waterbrash, and from time to time with heartburn.

The intestinal zone shows smaller and larger lacunae, from which a condition of digestive weakness is inferred. The widening of the iris-wreath in the temporal quadrant, including the large dilatations in the second minor zone, shows the likelihood of flatulence. The more or less strongly indicated white border of the intestinal zone (=iris-wreath) is a sign that the intestinal mucous membrane suffers from a state of chronic irritation.

On considering the iris-picture, it will be seen that there is generally a much lighter colouring for the kidney area in the second major zone, especially around the two small black signs at 31′ and 34′. At 29-31′ thick white bands extend from the second major zone into the gastro-intestinal zone and the first major zone is very much narrowed. Such signs when present invariably arise from the organ of the second major zone. In this case, a chronic inflammation of the kidney is shown, in which the small black signs indicate tissue damage. When such signs are seen, the urine should be examined (A).

The dark closed lacuna at 36-37′ in the second major zone is a sign for a resolved bladder condition (B). The dark sign immediately below, which deviates obliquely to the iris-rim, suggests that a condition of urethral discharge still exists. In this connection note the closed lacuna lying opposite at 5-7′ in the second major zone (C). This sign is suggestive of aortic aneurysm and is to be considered as being of hereditary origin, whereas the sign in Iris-4 indicated acquired infection.

The closed lacunae, which are seen generally distributed around the second major zone, are to be considered in relation to disturbances affecting the blood vessels. Even though the signs are placed in organ areas, one should first think of the blood vessels supplying those organs as well as of the blood itself.

Turning to the signs in sector 38-45′, apart from the closed lacuna at 43′ in the blood zone, there is also a small lacuna in the stomach zone at 42′, a larger lacuna in the intestinal zone at 41′ and a smaller lacuna in the blood zone at 40′. These three lacunae, lying obliquely one under the other, are each surrounded by a white border line (D). These signs have serious implications, especially in view of the oblique white lines and distorted black signs seen generally in this sector. The signs indicate severe disturbance of the nerve supply to the organs from lesions of the spinal vertebrae. In this context, the white flakes in the sixth minor zone are significant. They indicate inflammatory irritation of the lymphatic vessels and mucous membranes.

The scurf-rim in this sector (38-45′) is very dark and the white signs nowhere contact the iris-margin as they do in the remaining sectors. This indicates that the inflammatory activity is unable to diffuse outwards through the skin as elsewhere. Elimination through the skin is suppressed, whereas at other locations there may be irritating eruptions, either actual or latent.

The signs diametrically opposite at 7-12′ refer to the neck, including the atlas and cervical vertebrae (E). Corrective adjustment of vertebral lesions in the neck would support the medicinal treatment, ease the symptoms in the back and provide a positive influence to the stomach and urinary apparatus.

The grey-white deposit at the edge of the scurf-rim between 53′ and 10′, often described as a 'quicksilver-ring' is always a sign for scalp irritation (?—dissipation in youth) (F). This sign accords with the signs for bladder (37′), aorta (6′), ears (6′), kidney (30-33′) and back (40′). In addition, the large white sign at 26′ in the third major zone (gonads) should be taken into account.

Extract from the case record:

Patient 24 years of age, single, painter, the fourth child of four siblings.

Father died on active military service. Mother 60 years old and healthy.

No information concerning other antecedents.

Clinical features: finger nails short and flat; hair blonde, falling; complexion pallid, gaunt, yellowish skin; iris blue-grey. Irides of brothers and sisters—blue-grey.

History: In June 1938, developed an abscess over the left hip. In September 1938, fell down 8 metres and sustained injury to the head, legs and arms, especially affecting the left side. The tonsils were removed during childhood and at the age of 16 years the patient developed an inflammation of the hip-joint.

At the first consultation the patient complained of back pain, headaches and dizziness, and pain in the bladder and urethra. There was also a history of pressure over the epigastrium with eructations and severe abdominal flatulence. Because of the urogenital symptoms, the patient was referred for special treatment.

The stomach area (first minor zone) is readily seen as a light ring immediately around the pupil. The condition would not be regarded as involving any severe gastric disease, although here and there the outer margin is sharply demarcated, signifying a tendency to stomach cramp.

Looked at more closely, a wider black border is to be seen at the pupillary margin between 55´ and 10´. It appears as if the upper layer of the iris had been drawn back here, to expose the deepest pigmented layer at the edge of the pupil. At 2´ the condition is to be seen as a small projecting peak. These signs indicate disturbance affecting the central nervous system and in this case refer to attacks of migraine.

Likewise, the dark signs noted at the edge of the pupil at 28´, 37´ and 58´ are to be considered in the same connection. Their relation to other signs in the second and third major zones will be discussed later.

The dark colouring of the intestinal zone (second minor zone) is in contrast with the rest of the iris. The small and large lacunae show digestive weakness.

The radiating white lines (radials), some of which arise directly from the pupillary margin, traverse the intestinal zone and continue as far as the outer rim of the iris. Their presence suggests that intestinal colic occurs frequently. Note particularly that these white lines connect those organs which give rise to the migraine attacks: uterus, ovary and liver.

In this iris, there is a similar lightening of the kidney area (28´) to that seen in Iris-5, but with the difference that in Iris-6 no black signs are to be found. The white arc-line enclosing the large darkened area, which extends out to the third major zone, suggests a condition of floating kidney (A). Any kidney sign appearing in the right iris does not indicate so serious a condition as when the same sign appears in the left iris. Knowing this, and making a general comparison of the two irides, it may be said that not much can be promised to patient-5, especially in view of the deep heart sign at 16-17´ and the many black and white signs in the dorsal area between 38´ and 44´.

At 10-13´ in Iris-6 a darkened area is enclosed by two white lines which run together in an arc to the iris-wreath, thus forming an open lacuna. This sign suggests encumbrance of the pharynx and upper respiratory passages. The small closed lacuna immediately adjacent to the iris-wreath within this sign indicates involvement of the blood vascular system (B).

Note the sign formation at 41-45′ in the second and third major zones, diametrically opposite to that at 10-13′. The increased whiteness in the area shows that the lower air passages, bronchi and even the pleura are subject to chronic irritation. The signs at 15-20′ also accord with such a condition. The oblique white lines (transversals) indicate the presence of adhesions affecting the posterior pleural cavity. That some previous acute disturbance remains unresolved is shown not only by those signs so far described, but also by the very dark scurf-rim at 35-52′ which is so striking.

Now observe the oblique arc-lines (transversals) at 38-43′, which refer to a displaced sign for the liver (C). All signs for organ disturbances which are not normally seen in the lateral sectors of the iris, as with the liver sign here (38-43′) and the uterus sign (22-25′), but are displaced into those sectors, signify conditions which are difficult to influence.

The course of the iris-wreath in the areas for liver, lungs and pleura appears as a more or less straight line instead of the normal circular form. The displacement of the iris-wreath reflects the influence exerted upon the vegetative nervous system by such organs as the lungs, liver and kidneys. The white arc-lines at 29′, 27′, 40-45′ and 35′, which course from these last described signs in the second and third major zones inwards into the first major zone, almost as far as the pupillary margin, indicate that the disturbances are connected with the central nervous system. On close examination, the black lines radiating from the pupillary margin will be seen.

The sign for the uterus, which is not readily apparent, may now be explained further. Apart from pressure downwards and on the rectum, the abdominal symptoms are not severe. The somewhat loosened structure of the radial fibres seen between two thick white lines: one commencing at 29′ at the iris-wreath and extending obliquely to the iris-rim at 26′, and the other commencing at 21′ at the iris-wreath and extending as an arc to 23′ on the iris-rim, suggest that the uterus is enlarged and displaced posteriorly (D).

Diametrically opposite at 55′ in the third minor zone, a closed lacuna is seen adjacent to the iris-wreath, as well as a dark sign in the fourth and fifth minor zones (E). This last sign is actually a red pigment fleck (toxin-sign), while the lacuna should be regarded as the result of the abdominal condition.

The interpretation of these signs as the cause of the migraine attacks should not be taken to mean that similar signs would be present in every patient suffering from migraine. In this connection the following singular case illustrates the principle involved: A large and well-nourished man came to me for consultation. After the iris examination it was explained to him among other things that he was suffering from gall-stones. His reply was that apart from stomach symptoms he had felt nothing of gall-stones. What most gave him discomfort was migraine and he could drink neither alcohol nor beer if he did not want to be completly incapable of work on the following day because of headache. These attacks had already persisted for a long time and were becoming progressively worse. I did not depart from my diagnosis, but advised him that when he was free of biliary stasis and gall-stones, he would also be free of migraine.

In spite of his doubts about the diagnosis he promised to take the prescribed medicine. After fourteen days he returned and reported that he had meanwhile suffered a severe attack of biliary colic and that the attending physician had confirmed the existence of gall-stones. A second prescription was now given together with dietetic advice, but which as a travelling business man he was unable to follow. By the third visit the patient reported that he had suffered no further attacks of colic or migraine, although several days before he had become rather inebriated.

To return to Iris-6: extract from the case record—
Housewife, 40 years of age, married with one child, the second child of five siblings. One brother died from intestinal tuberculosis at the age of 19 years.
The patient's father died at the age of 46 years from lung disease (stone-cutters pneumoconiosis). The mother was still living, 62 years of age and healthy. The paternal grandfather died from asthma at the age of 72 years. The paternal grandmother died very early in childbirth. The maternal grandfather died from cancer at the age of 52 years and the maternal grandmother died in childbirth.

35

Clinical findings: nails short and domed; hair dark blonde; complexion ruddy.

Past history: measles at 20 years of age, diphtheria at 24 years of age, a bladder-mole had been removed and during the second pregnancy an open tubercular ulcer of the bone affected the left great toe. A rupture of the left lung following over-exertion occurred at the age of 37 years. Stomach symptoms had been present from 28 years of age and the patient had been treated for gastric ulcers. After an accident to the thorax involving fracture of ribs, the right breast shrunk. Severe attacks of migraine had persisted for some years.

At the first consultation the patient had complained of heart symptoms with pains radiating down into the left hand. Vertex pressure and pain in the head, stomach and intestinal symptoms with flatulence, periodic attacks of severe migraine and a tendency to melancholia, were also noted.

Iris-7   **Female: 25 years—left iris**

In this case the pupil is too large, and the vertical elliptic shape suggests nervous weakness. The nerve ring (pupillary margin) is too dark, indicating portal congestion. Note the dark radiations from the pupil, especially the organ areas to which the black peaks point. In those organs the complaints are likely to be found. These signs indicate participation of the central nervous system.

The stomach area is very white, and is readily seen as a bright ring. There is an increased production of stomach acid, giving rise to heartburn. Several locations in the stomach area, especially from 50′ to 5′ and at 32′, show a more severe condition and involve inflammation of the stomach wall with increased pain.

The area for large intestine (second minor zone) shows a white iris-wreath with large dilatations, indicating a pathological state of the colon. A severe condition of unresolved catarrh in youth has become a chronic state of the intestine.

In the lower part of the descending colon at 25′, several small weakness signs are to be seen lying somewhat obliquely. In the large lacuna extending over the blood and muscle zones (third and fourth minor zones) similar signs are also to be found. Such signs indicate a weakness of the wall of the intestine with a tendency to perforation. In this case, perforation may be presumed already in view of the chronic inflammation of the peritoneum as shown by the white signs in the third major zone at 22-28', which extend as far as the iris rim. I find these last signs more or less strongly indicated whenever perforation of the intestine has occurred. After some years, anal fistulae or a gravitation abscess of the thigh may develop.

The markedly white signs in the area for rectum (second and third major zones) at 37' and 38' should also be considered in this context. Where the white signs in the sixth minor zone extend as far as the iris-rim in the shape of bundles, such skin affections as itching, burning and eruptions may be anticipated. The three dark lines in the area for rectum at 37' in the third major zone, together with the white lines extending to the iris-rim, are signs for burning and itching of the anus with secretion of mucous.

According to the case history the following symptoms were complained of at the time the photograph was taken: Frequent occurrence of diarrhoea with blood, together with heavy haemorrhages from the bowel. Disposition to take cold easily and a poor state of the blood. According to the statements of the doctors, the intestinal bleeding was coming from a higher part of the colon and was not simply haemorrhoidal bleeding.

A dark brown 'neurasthenic' ring (pupillary margin) indicates portal congestion and is associated with rectal conditions (haemorrhoids). This connection should be noted, for even though there may be no possible scientific justification, yet in relation to the symptoms it will be found confirmed.

The large dark closed and open lacunae observed in this iris show considerable general weakness. From the signs in the first major zone, where the organs of food preparation are shown, it is apparent that there is insufficient processing of nutritional materials, with the consequence that toxic substances are absorbed to encumber and weaken the organs of metabolic activity. These lacunae extend as far out as the fifth minor zone (bone zone). The area for the mucous membranes is at the junction with the sixth minor zone, showing an almost total ring of white flakes in the form of a garland (lymphatic rosary). The thick white lines extending from the iris-wreath to the outer ring of white flakes (lymph vascular system—'lymph-bridges') portray the connection between the over-burdened mucous membranes and the organs of food preparation (stomach and intestines). Patients showing these iris signs are generally stout and bloated, without power or endurance. They are unable to readjust their way of life and since they are also unaware of the extent of the problem they never have time for a complete resolution of the condition.

Now to the signs in detail: Remaining with the white signs, which always indicate acute inflammation or painful conditions, it will be noticed that those signs from 13′ to 16′ and from 34′ to 38′ show a lighter tone than elsewhere and are relatively closer to the iris-wreath. This indicates that the organs reflected in those sectors have been subjected to chronic irritation for a long time (13-16′ = heart and lungs, 34-38′ = rectum and bladder). If it is also established from the case history that there was asthma on the father's side and tuberculosis on the mother's side affecting the antecedents, then it may be assumed that there will be a tendency to sexual irritation in the patient.

However, over-stimulation of the sexual organs arises not only from hereditary influences, but also from disturbance of the digestive organs. This can also be seen in the iris. The large dark lacuna at 25-28′ in the area for ovary (A) is not only the consequence of the present state of the large intestine, but taken together with the signs at 37′ and 38′ (bladder area) suggests that the patient is subject to masturbation. This accords with the indications of the large dark lacuna seen in the area for arm (B) and the long narrow lacuna seen in the diametrically opposite sector (mouth area) (C), signifying taciturnity and silent withdrawal.

The large lacunae in the dorsal area (40-45′) suggest weakness of the spinal cord in general and are signs for a tubercular tendency. The signs in the brain area at 55-5′ are obscured so that any indications relative to the foregoing conditions cannot be given.

There remains the small closed lacuna at 28′, close to the iris-wreath (D), which indicates disturbance of the suprarenal function and secondarily of the vegetative nervous system (autonomic dystony). The open lacuna with a thick white border at 40-42′ in the second major zone is a sign for the pancreas. (E) The closed lacuna at 22-23′ in the second major zone also refers to the pancreas and is here displaced to a lower position as a result of the enlarged first major zone (F), indicating ptosis and displacement. This latter sign should raise the question of a possible diabetes and even if there is as yet no evidence of glycosuria, the patient should be so informed and given directions concerning diet. In patients showing these signs nutrition is always faulty: they live too well and especially eat too much fatty food and sweet things.

Iris-8   Male 53 years—left iris

On this picture the pupillary margin cannot be seen. Such a condition indicates that there is severe involvement of the central nervous system in which the reactive capacity is very weak or hardly present at all. This is especially evident from the rather black striations seen in the stomach area which begin at the pupil. In this case, a severe deterioration of the gastric mucous membrane may be assumed, and the white mottled appearance of the outer border of the stomach area is a sign for inflammatory involvement of the muscle layer of the stomach.

Signs for rheumatic inflammation are to be found in the intestinal zone (second minor zone), especially at 8-10′, 32-38′, 48-52′ and 55-60′. Here there is a gastro-intestinal disturbance which is aggravated by every change of the weather. However, since the whole iris is covered with signs indicating rheumatic conditions, a situation can occur in which the rheumatic pains elsewhere can be so severe as to mask the stomach symptoms. In most cases the secretion of gastric juice is disturbed and the patient complains of occasional burning sensation in the stomach which, as with peptic ulcer, is improved by eating. But at times the pains suddenly disappear and then just as suddenly reappear. If the stomach zone is considered more closely, small black dots will be seen at many places. These signs are to be regarded as indicating ulcerous processes.

The intestinal zone (second minor zone) shows several peaked dilatations, suggesting a background of faulty nutrition. More particularly striking is the peak at 42′, a sign that the pains are concentrated in the back between the shoulder blades. The white transversal, seen as an oblique line in the intestinal zone, which proceeds outwards from the border of the intestinal area to the iris-rim, indicates the presence of adhesions affecting the small intestine and giving rise to severe pains in that region. The large intestinal peak at 54′ pointing towards the forehead region suggests the presence of frontal pains.

The following details are recorded on the case card:

Mother, 76 years old, has always suffered from stomach symptoms. Father died from pneumonia at the age of 78 years.

The patient is 53 years of age and has always suffered with gastric disturbances.

In this patient there is a hereditary tendency to stomach disorders, which in the mother were probably based on a rheumatic diathesis, so it is not surprising that severe disturbances should arise in a man working in a humid atmosphere. He has been under treatment previously for gastroptosis and gastric ulcer.

This iris well illustrates the existing acute phase of rheumatism. In relation to rheumatic patients generally, almost every practitioner nowadays thinks of suprarenal disturbance or cortisone insufficiency. Indeed, to the irisdiagnostician the concept is familiar, but only when a suprarenal sign exists in the iris would it be agreed. If such is not the case, then cortisone will have no influence and its therapeutic use will fail.

If, as here, a sign is seen diametrically opposite at 57-58', the pituitary area, then it will be found that cortisone medication is effective only for so long as it is given and that on withdrawal of the medication the old condition returns and may even be worse. (A)

The pituitary function controls all the glands of internal secretion and where it is disturbed, either there is obstruction to the restorative action of cortisone or an accentuation of its effect. However, with such a condition of suprarenal function as is shown by the iris-sign here (B), there will be a secondary influence affecting the vegetative nervous system involving vaso-contraction and circulatory disturbance. As a consequence, the supply of blood and nutrition to organs and tissues is reduced and focal infection arises. This, in turn, produces circulatory stress, systemic dysfunction and ultimately leads to general breakdown.

In patients showing a similar iris-pattern, note especially the presence of prominent radials, commencing either at the pupillary margin or the iris-wreath and extending outwards to the iris-rim, as well as shining white clouds. The organ areas in which these signs appear will mark the focus of the chief complaints. The small, dark, point-like signs, distributed generally over the iris, merit particular attention, since they indicate insufficiency of lymph-node activity as the consequence of an over-stressed lymphatic system from toxic saturation.

40

In such conditions the development of glandular swellings (cold ulcers) and caseous degeneration may easily follow. Inflammation and oxidation in the tissues and joints with consequent rheumatic pain is the attempt by the organism to help itself.

Now observe the point-like signs at 46-47′, 49′ and 51-52′ in the fifth and sixth minor zones, indicating that the patient suffers from bleeding gums and has suppurative foci at the roots of the teeth. In that sector of the scleral conjunctival mucous membrane adjacent to the iris area for maxilla and nasal sinus at 47-49′, prominent blood vessels are seen. This configuration suggests that the area is the subject of raised vital activity from increased blood supply (hyperaemia). A small bluish point seen at the end of the branching blood vessel indicates the presence of some non-disseminating focus, e.g. dormant granuloma.

The dark sign at 40-42′ in the fourth and fifth minor zones, contains a small black point (C). The black point is, in fact, a fault on the photographic plate and has no significance, but the dark sign as such shows disturbance of the spinal cord. Unlike the lacunae seen at 26-33′, which extend from the iris-wreath to the iris-rim as long signs, it begins only in the muscle zone and ends at the inner border of the scurf-rim (sixth minor zone) as short radials, thus showing a greater transverse width. This fact suggests that there is an ulcerous process exerting pressure to force the tissues apart. Similarly with the suprarenal sign at 28′ (B), an enlargement is suggested. However, since there are no oblique lines at the sign at 40′, there is no suggestion of injury. The prominent white radials which traverse the sign and extend from the iris-wreath to the iris-rim show the presence of painful conditions.

The presence of dense white clouds in close proximity to the dark signs at 39′ and 43′ suggests inflammatory irritation of the adjacent tissues. Also consider the prominent white border surrounding the suprarenal sign (B). This patient had a large fatty tumour, the size of the fist, situated on the left side of the lower lumbar vertebrae, which was causing pressure symptoms. However, the rheumatic symptoms are in the foreground of all complaints.

Iris photographs 9 and 10 are the left and right eyes of the same patient. The pupil has the shape of a vertical ellipse similar to that in illustration No. 7.

The stomach zone (first minor zone) is on the whole too large, especially in relation to the intestinal zone. This is a sign for dilatation of the stomach. The white outer border of the stomach ring at 42-52' suggests inflammation of the muscle layer. In addition, white blobs are to be seen within the stomach area, especially between 15' and 25', which indicate rheumatic irritation of the stomach muscle.

The intestinal zone (second minor zone) is generally speaking too small in comparison with the stomach zone. The presence of a white line at sections of the iris-wreath suggests chronic intestinal catarrh with a tendency to shrinking. Several small black points are to be seen at 35-55' in the area for small intestine towards the edge of the second minor zone. These are indications of defect signs (ulcer signs), although there may not be any remaining active ulceration. (A)

In my view, the presence of such intestinal signs indicates that the intestinal glands were inflamed at some time during childhood. Passing undetected at the time, the glands became indurated and subsequently atrophied. Consequently, damaged areas of the intestinal mucous membrane may arise which can lead to all kinds of conditions. Intestinal erosions and adhesions are here evidenced by the signs at 31', 42-45', 47' and 55', where the white line of the iris-wreath is interrupted.

A flattening of the intestinal zone in the upper quadrant of the iris is a sign for ptosis of the transverse colon. The considerable widening of the second minor zone from 4' to 15', including the two peaks, indicates distension of the left (splenic) flexure of the colon. The sharp indentation of the zone which follows indicates contraction or constriction. (B)

Since this widened section encroaches upon the area for the heart at 15' (third minor zone) it suggests that heart complaints would arise from flatulent distension, expressing as symptoms of cardiac oppression and palpitation (Roemheld syndrome).

At 10' in the first major zone, commencing at the iris-wreath, a white line is to be seen running towards the pupillary margin

(= transversal). Somewhat higher, a transversal is also indicated. These show the presence of adhesions. (B)

Referring to the dorsal region (40-45′), several small black signs located in the fourth and fifth minor zones (muscle/bone) are to be seen at 42′. They are defect-signs, and in this case represent old injuries. From the uppermost black sign a fine white line runs out obliquely to terminate at the outer border of the iris at 37′ (= adhesion/injury sign). These signs indicate that there must have been some old injury to the spine or the coccyx as from a fall. However, the white clouds in the fifth and sixth minor zones adjacent to the dark sign at 42′ suggest a persistent acute inflammation. The elongated white sign going out from the iris-wreath at 43′, and the small white clouds at 45′, are to be considered in connection with the signs at 42′. (C)

I explained to the patient that she must have suffered earlier from an injury to the back which had resulted in inflammation of the dorsal vertebrae and the production of severe pains. After confirmation by the patient, I advised attendance at the orthopaedic department of the local medical clinic for radiographic examination and treatment. The patient later informed me that my diagnosis had been confirmed and that long-term treatment was required.

The sign originating at the iris-wreath and extending to the outer border of the iris (23-27′) suggests a persistent inflammation of the uterine adnexa. The white cloud at 25-26′ in the third major zone indicates that inflammatory irritation of the ovary is present. In this rheumatic disposition and potential tuberculosis, any condition of suffering affecting an organ is to be regarded as tubercular. (D) Case card: Housewife, 32 years, one child. Symptoms declared at the first consultation: stomach pains and feeling of fulness, sour eructations and frequent diarrhoea, pain on micturition and discharge.

History: 1926—severe influenza. 1930—curettage on account of severe haemorrhage. 1931—fall on to the back. Back pain has developed since that time and has recently become increasingly worse. No details of antecedents.

Iris-10   **Female: 32 years—right iris**

The photographs 9 and 10 are the right and left eyes of the same patient. As with the left eye, the right pupil has the shape of a vertical ellipse. The explanation given concerning the relative sizes of the stomach and intestinal zones and the background rheumatoid condition also applies.

The black striation of the first minor zone in the right iris signifies a hereditary predisposition to diseases of the stomach and intestines. In the pyloric area of the stomach zone at 15', three large punctate irregularly shaped signs are to be seen lying closely together, one under the other and surrounded by a white colouring. The black punctate signs indicate ulcerous processes, while the white colouring suggests inflammation. Thus, the acute phase of ulceration has not yet completely receded, and the pyloric ulcers are still active. (A)

In the first minor zone at 42-45', four black elongated signs are to be found lying one under the other. The uppermost and largest sign is still active whereas the remaining lesions can be already closed. However, the inflammatory character persists in all locations, including those at 15', as denoted by the strongly white colouring of the surrounding area. (White colouring and white flakes are signs for inflammation) (B)

Consider the small black sign in the intestinal zone (second minor zone) at 40', which begins in the first minor zone. This sign is separated from an adjacent small black sign by an oblique white stroke and indicates the presence of a duodenal ulcer with scar tissue formation (C). Just below this there are two small black signs within the intestinal zone with another two black points immediately outside the iris-wreath. These four signs are to be considered together, and indicate the presence of adhesions following active ulceration affecting the first part of the duodenum. That this location still has a strongly inflammatory character is seen in the intensely white colouring of the locality. The presence of pain is denoted by the wavy radiating white lines which arise in the stomach zone and course outwards to the iris-rim. The course of these lines is especially striking, since the lineation is far from clear and the course very disturbed.

From the fourth minor zone outwards, the white lines enclose a long almost black sign which extends as far as the iris-rim. This sign indicates that the gall ducts are affected by adhesions. Swelling of the liver is suggested by the darker area at the iris-rim extending from 37' to 43' and enclosed by an arc-shaped white line. The dark sign at 39-40′ in the fourth minor zone (muscle zone) enclosing a black point in the centre and a small black stroke at the lower edge, is to be regarded as a gall-bladder sign (D).

The diagnosis is: biliary stasis from displacement of the bile duct, gall stone formation and swelling of the liver, arising from duodenal ulceration. Apart from the presence of stomach pains and a feeling of fullness with bitter eructations, the first consultation included a complaint of severe back pain.

The remarks made under Iris-9 concerning the size of the first major zone and the white line at the iris-wreath, also apply to this iris. In the small intestine area, between 5′ and 35′ in the second minor zone, the number of black points is fewer than in the left iris (25-55′). Several small black lacunae lying one under the other can be seen at 10-15′ in the intestinal zone, showing an atrophic condition of the muscle layer. In the area for caecum and appendix, at 36′ in the second minor zone, a dark rhomboid-shaped sign with its outer point breaking through the iris-wreath and from which a white wavy line courses outward to the iris-rim, suggests the existence of adhesions affecting the caecal area (E). Indeed, the whole region of the ascending colon is affected by adhesions, as shown by the confused delineation of the fibres in the third minor zone from 36′ to 40′. Also, the transversal appearing in the sixth minor zone between 36′ and 39′ suggests that an operation upon the appendix has been undertaken (E).

The large peaked dilatation of the intestinal area at 50′ is a sign for flatulent distension and intestinal colic, leading to a high position of the diaphragm with consequent symptoms of oppression and shortness of breath (Roemheld). This condition is to be considered together with the dropped transverse colon, signs for which are less striking than those in the left iris (Iris-9). (F)

Note the dark sign at 42-45′ in the third and fourth minor zones (blood and muscle zones). This sign is a lacuna in the area for bronchi, the lower border of which is a straight line running obliquely from the iris-wreath and giving a generally downward inclination to the whole sign. Thus, an organ displacement is indicated and probably arises from the pressure of an enlarged liver and the effect of large intestine distension upon the diaphragm (G).

The dark sign at 45-48′, which begins in the muscle zone, shows weakness of the lung tissue and suggests that the antecedents suffered from pulmonary disease. A similar sign is more frequently seen after unresolved whooping cough, especially when, as here, there is also a bronchial sign. In this case, the iris-rim (skin zone) is very dark, showing suppressed conditions. The patient confirmed that the antecedents had suffered from asthma and that in youth she had developed severe whooping cough which left a susceptibility to cough with expectoration. (H)

The existence of this weakness is confirmed by the white flakes seen in the fourth and fifth minor zones at 45', 48' and 50', together with the small white flakes at 11' and 13' in the same zones and showing small, long, dark signs between (Mouth and throat area).

The oblique formation of small dark/black signs lying one above the other at 15-16' in the fourth and fifth minor zones, which continues in an upward and outward direction to 14', is suggestive of upward displacement of the radial white lines. The question of spinal vertebral displacement arises. However, the cause lies more deeply, at 17-18', where a small black point is to be seen just above the prominent white radial which extends from the iris-wreath to the outer border (J).

The white zig-zag lines to be seen at 15-20' in the dorsal area indicate that severe pains affect this region. These last described signs concerning the dorsal area must be completed by assessing the signs in the left iris.

The dark wedge-sign at 23-25', with its base to the iris-wreath and its peak in the fifth minor zone, includes a black-brown toxin-fleck and has a small black point within the peak. This sign is in the bladder area. The small black sign at 28' at the iris-wreath refers to the kidney (K). These signs taken together suggest that there is a hereditary condition affecting the urinary apparatus, as is also the case with the lung signs. When such conditions affect the bladder, it will be found that treatment does not readily achieve results.

Iris-11   **Female: 30 years—right iris**

In this case, the shape of the pupil should be ignored, since as with the iris, it arises from the oblique position of the eyes while being photographed.

The whole stomach area (first minor zone) appears very white, indicating a severe degree of inflammation. Pain in the stomach and abdomen with sour belching occurs upon the slightest dietetic error. At 11′ and 15′ (pylorus), 40-43′ and 45-53′, large elongated dark streaks and lacunae are seen extending from the pupil to the iris-wreath. These signs indicate the presence of adhesions following ulcerative processes. The more intensely white area in the stomach zone at 42′ and 57′ shows the persistence of a more severe degree of inflammation (A). The many indentations and sharp peaks seen in the second minor zone (iris-wreath) suggest the occurrence of severe attacks of colic affecting the small and large intestine.

The small elongated black sign lying in the white iris-wreath at 35′ (caecal area) merits special attention. Inflammation of the appendix with suppuration has occurred here. The enclosed black sign indicates loss of tissue substance through ulcerative processes, while the intensely white surrounding shows chronic inflammation. In this connection, several black signs in the ciliary zones should be noted. The first sign is just outside the iris-wreath at 36′ in the blood zone, the second in the muscle zone and the third in the third major zone. This last sign is larger and actually consists of several small black points and lines. These signs indicate that the suppurative inflammation has extended to the peritoneum (B).

Still in relation to this same condition, note the white oblique lines in the third major zone from 34′ to 38′ (transversals). Even though these lines are broken and not particularly striking, the diagnosis must be: chronic inflammation of the appendix with adhesions to the peritoneum. Whether or not an operation has taken place must be decided from the interrogation of the patient (B). These oblique white lines (transversals) may also arise after an operation, but if no operation has been undertaken so far, then on the appearance of persistent pain the patient should be referred immediately for surgical treatment. If, however, an operation has been carried out already and pain still persists, then such a condition is very difficult to treat.

The duodenal signs at 40-43′ in the second minor zone are to be considered together with the large lacuna, which beginning at 48′ in the stomach zone, breaks through the iris-wreath to continue as a white line extending as far as the muscle zone. Since small black signs are seen to be enclosed, then adhesions to the duodenum are affecting the colon below the right (hepatic) flexure (C).

The strongly indented iris-wreath at 29′ and 31′, opposite the sectors for kidney and suprarenal gland, should also be considered in this context. But at the same time, the wreath indications, together with the signs in the renal and suprarenal areas, show disturbances of the organs themselves. (D).

On the case record is noted: No information concerning the father. The mother died from pulmonary tuberculosis at the age of 40 years. The patient is 30 years old. As a child she suffered severely from scrofulous enlargement of the glands and also had measles. She was variously treated for stomach illness over 10 years. At 27 years of age, radiographic examination indicated chronic inflammation with adhesions in the caecal area. On the second consultation, acute inflammation with adhesions in the caecal area was evident and the patient was referred for immediate surgical treatment. At the operation it was found that there were infective foci in addition to severe adhesions in the region of the appendix. The operation lasted for three hours. The iris photograph was taken before the operation.

Considering the iris generally outside the first major zone, it will be seen that it is full of open and closed lacunae, some of which extend to the iris-rim. Being in the right iris, these signs indicate long standing conditions of hereditary weakness.

What is the basis for these conditions? The hereditary tubercular disposition is to be seen in the large lacunae positioned respectively at 7-14' (mouth and throat), 45-50' (lungs), and 15-20' (pleura, back). In these sectors the iris-wreath is displaced inwards as far as the first minor zone, showing that the related vegetative nerve centres are disturbed. This autonomic disturbance is especially apparent in the sectors for kidney and suprarenal gland where the wreath line reaches the pupillary margin (E). (Iris-wreath = vegetative nervous system; pupillary margin = central nervous system).

Further to these signs, consider the lacunae at 59-60' in the area for midbrain and at 3-4' in the area for pituitary gland (diametrically opposite respectively to the signs for kidney and suprarenal gland). (F) From these signs it is evident that the weakness involves the endocrine system and the mid-brain with its mento-emotional connections. The lacunae at 40' (pancreas) and 25' (bladder) are also in accordance with this state.

If in such cases, signs for kidney and suprarenal gland are seen in the left iris, with nothing apparent in the lung area, there may yet be an early condition of tuberculosis to be considered.

48

The seeming displacement of the first major zone should raise the question of a possible abdominal tumour. With the chronic disturbances in the abdominal cavity and the present suppurative conditions, a cystic development could easily arise from the right ovary, but probably this could only be ascertained by surgical investigation.

Iris-12   **Male: 27 years—right iris**

The pupil is too small and indicates hypersensibility of the nervous system. The stomach zone (first minor zone) is seen as a large white circle. However, this could not be described as indicating enlargement of the stomach. More detailed observation reveals the presence of white wedge signs between 15' and 25' and from 32' to 40' (A). Thus there exists a condition of high acid production with inflammation extending to the tissues surrounding the stomach. This intense hyperacidity is not due to rheuma, but has arisen from too much carbohydrate food and insufficient mastication (lack of salivary digestion). The resultant hyper-alimentation syndrome is the consequence of excessive carbohydrate and produces the triad of symptoms: meteorism, heartburn and coronary symptoms. There is little prospect of cure.

The intestinal area (second minor zone), especially that between 8' and 35', shows signs of worse conditions than those of the large intestine area between 35' and 38', and indicates that such conditions are difficult to heal, being the consequence of the syndrome described above. To be noted more especially are the two wedge-signs which can be traced inwards from the outer iris-rim as far as the stomach zone. The upper limb of the first wedge-sign proceeds from 6' at the iris-rim obliquely downwards to intersect the border of the stomach zone. This sign, consisting of an inward deviation of the second minor zone, obscures the intestinal area. It is not a sign for intestine disease, but points to severe conditions affecting the organs in the outer zones of the iris (B). The same applies in the case of the second wedge-sign at 24-30', indicating severe disturbance of the kidney (C).

The outward bulging of the area for large intestine, and the large and small lacunae with their surrounding white borders, indicate conditions which are to be ascribed to severe damage from faulty nutrition and unresolved conditions during infancy.

Case history:
Profession painter, 27 years of age. Has been under medical treatment for the past year. The stomach pains are precipitated by chill. Severe stomach pains with considerable burning and sour eructations occur. The burning sensation extends up into the mouth. The pains improve after drinking hot fluids (note the homoeopathic rule: heat for heat). In addition, there is a condition of back pain with insomnia.

The only brother of the father died at the age of 46 years from cancer of the stomach. Otherwise, there was no special hereditary encumbrance.

Consideration of the iris findings shows that the patient must be extremely careful of his stomach. It would be beneficial to re-examine the patient several times each year, since all his complaints will have their origin in the conditions of stomach and intestines.

The effect of the disorders of stomach and intestines upon other organs of the body may now be considered. The wedge-sign at 6-13′, covering the area for mouth and naso-pharynx, which displaces the iris-wreath inwards to peak at 11′ in the stomach zone, indicates that the local vegetative nerve centre is affected (B). Such a sign denotes the existence of conditions which would be difficult to heal and the symptoms which are now present, or are yet to appear, would not be readily influenced.

In these areas are to be found not merely the small lacunae, but all degrees of pathology, from signs of inflammation (white clouds), to indications of tissue breakdown (dark to black wisp signs), and ultimately to evidence of dessication and atrophy (dark to black signs intersected by small white lines) (B). Overall, it is the picture for chronic catarrh of the maxillary sinuses, extending to encroach upon the naso-pharynx, larynx and trachea. The mucous membranes are inflamed, broken down and suppurating, and already show the tendency to atrophy.

The white lines running obliquely across the area (transversals) are also to be found in the whole of the outer zones of the iris. They appear especially striking at 44-55′ in the fifth minor zone, probably because of the reduced intensity of inflammation signs compared with the areas 15-25′ and 30-41′, the former being due to the encumbrance of the vertebral column and the severe involvement of the small intestine, and the latter to the condition of the peritoneum, the caecum and the colon.

The wedge-sign in the area 24-30' is similar to that in the neck area and with its thick white border indicates a condition of persistent renal catarrh following inflammation of the kidney (C).

Consider now the dark sign at 38-41' adjacent to the iris-wreath and extending into the muscle zone (fourth minor zone) (D). How does this extension arise and what does it signify? This sign, located in the area for pancreas, suggests the existence of swelling of the organ with functional insufficiency. The two black dots located within the outer edge of the sign indicate tissue defects (loss of substance) within the pancreas.

This situation probably arises from adhesions following inflammation of the duodenum, which can be recognised by the small dark lacunae and the thick white oblique lines in the areas for pylorus and duodenum in the gastro-intestinal zone (D). As already stated, inflammation of the kidney can involve contiguous organs pathologically and as in this case, give rise to adhesions affecting the duodenum and colon. It is probably here, that renal inflammation developed in early youth and provided the basis for the sign complex in this area.

The markedly wide and dark iris-rim and the white flakes at 48-50' indicate that acute catarrhal conditions such as colds and influenza have been suppressed. The widening of the dark iris-rim from 38' to 43' suggests a condition of stasis of the liver accompanied by some slight swelling. As a result of the adhesions affecting the duodenum there would be obstruction to the discharge of pancreatic secretion and bile with consequent enlargement of the liver and pancreas.

One aspect should again be stressed: in the area between 13' and 40' there is marked discoloration of the iris from heavy white deposits extending outwards as far as the iris-rim. From this it may be deduced that the organs covered by these deposits are the subject of increased vital activity as the organism endeavours to eliminate the encumbrance through the skin. In cases where the white deposits extend as far as the outer rim of the iris, it can be assumed that skin eruptions represent systemic elimination and interrogation of the patient will usually produce confirmation of their existence. If this should not be the case, it usually needs no more than some alterative medication to produce the reaction.

However, in this respect note the differences of natural colour. The white appearance observed in a black and white picture may represent any shade from brightest white to reddish-brown. From the natural colour, the duration of the condition in the lymph-vascular system and the origin of the material may be recognised. The longer the condition exists, the darker the deposits will appear. If they appear white, then an acute inflammatory disturbance is present. Conditions which stem from excessive intake of carbohydrate will either remain white or turn grey. If the deposits become brownish, then the condition has its origin in fat or protein poisoning.

The background of this sign-complex may be interpreted as follows: the over-consumption of carbohydrate (sugar) produces inflammation of the gastro-intestinal mucous membrane from which white signs appear in the iris. The secondary consequence of this is the development of inflammatory reaction affecting the lymph-vascular (lacteal) system of the intestine, which in turn extends to encroach upon the whole lymph-vascular system of the organism.

But carbohydrate is not the only cause of such conditions, fat is probably even more dangerous. Fats are decomposed in the duodenum into fatty acid and glycerine. The fatty acid requires emulsification with bile in order that transudation through the mucous membrane may be made. If because of excessive intake of fat and relative insufficiency of bile this does not take place, then the glycerine is absorbed from the intestine, and in the absence of fatty acid constitutes an injurious material which initiates inflammation of the intestinal mucosa.

Under these conditions the mucous membrane becomes permeable to foreign proteins which constitute a severe toxin when circulating in the blood. This poisonous material is eliminated from the blood by the activity of the phagocytes, which after absorption of the toxin, migrate into the lymphatic system. The increased vital reactivity of this system gives rise to the white colouring of the iris-wreath and this extends over the intermediate blood and muscle zones to the outer areas. If in chronic conditions light to dark-brown deposits are seen in the iris, then these are signs for damage from protein products.

From these photographs it can be seen immediately that there is a severe condition of the stomach and intestines.

The pupillary ring is flattened in several locations, from which appearance the state of the central nervous system is recognised as being very poor.

The dark signs in the stomach area (first minor zone), at 30′ and 37-40′ in the right iris next to the pupillary margin, are suggestive of cancer.

The large white indentation at 37′ right iris (second minor zone) shows inflammatory adhesions in the caecal area, and the black spot in this area indicates loss of tissue from a suppurative process. The numerous transversals in the third major zone between 30′ and 38′ in the right iris also indicate many adhesions (A).

The inward deviation of the iris-wreath at 33′ in the right iris, with the black rhomboid sign at the outer border in the third minor zone, is a suprarenal sign (B).

The small and large dark signs which lie in the widened area of the intestinal ring between 37′ and 54′ right iris, are signs for ulceration and adhesions affecting the duodenum and large intestine. Diametrically opposite, in the area for small intestine at 13-23′, similar signs for ulceration are to be seen.

The wedge-sign at 17-22′ in the right iris, with its peak pointing outwards, is especially serious. It is formed from oblique white lines (transversals). This sign encloses the signs for adhesions affecting the posterior wall of the stomach, the duodenum and pancreas (C).

In the left iris (No. 14) note the wedge sign between 35′ and 40′ with its base in the stomach zone and its peak in the third major zone (D). This sign indicates that the tail of the pancreas is already affected by adhesions, giving rise to slight glycosuria and confirming the presumptive condition of diabetes mellitus.

In the same context, consider in both irides the intensely white signs for inflammation in the stomach and intestinal zones, as well as outside the gastro-intestinal area. Such signs indicate that the condition is already very far advanced.

The principal painful conditions may be located by noting where the white radial fibres are thickened and agglomerated, running outwards from the pupil to the iris-rim and breaking through the sclerotic ring. This ring, which at the age of 39 years already appears so prominent, is a sign for an early demise.

The large lacunae at 45-52' in the lung area of the right iris, together with the lacunae at 40-45' (chest and bronchi) and the signs at 8-15' (mouth, pharynx and trachea) suggest the possibility of a tubercular tendency, which in fact exists as a hereditary predisposition. In this connection note the large dark lacunae in the areas for the respiratory organs in both iris pictures, from which the tubercular encumbrance is evident. The small kidney sign at 31-33' in the left iris at the iris-wreath (Iris-14) is also to be regarded as a tubercular sign (E).

However, in spite of the above evidence, how does it arise that a cancerous condition should be considered? Note the small grey gastro-intestinal zone with the grey-black signs. Such signs always indicate a tendency to atrophy and induration. By comparison, the texture in the second and third major zones is generally looser, the white radial lines coarser and with the spaces between wider and darker. Moreover, the dark lacunae in the organ areas are not so oval but extend as far as the iris-margin. The iris thus acquires a grey discolouration (the 'combed-hair' of Maubach).

In this respect compare Iris-7. The inflammatory state of the lymphatic tissues to be seen in this iris is replaced in Iris-13 and Iris-14 by the arcus senilis, which also portrays atrophy and induration of the tissues. Now note the scar formation at 37-40' of the second and third major zones in the right iris (Iris-13), and compare these signs with the signs in the same area of Iris-24. It will be apparent that the same sign formation which is so strongly presented in Iris-24 is in the early stages of formation in Iris-13.

Likewise with the flattening of the iris-rim at 35-40' of right iris-13. However, it should not be thought that every cancerous condition develops as slowly as is the case with the patients whose irides are shown in illustrations 13, 14 and 24. These are patients in whom a chronic condition of the stomach has resulted in a gradual induration and atrophy of the tissues. The irritation from the thick scar-tissue formation, arising from an earlier ulcerated condition, results in tumour formation and ultimate destructive pathology.

There is yet another consideration in the development of a cancerous condition. It is to be remembered with patients who suddenly develop stomach symptoms after apparently good health (in spite of long over-eating) and within three months are dead from cancer. In these cases the iris will show encumbrance of the lymphatic system and a large gastro-intestinal ring (first major zone). However, the obvious weakness signs are never found, as in Iris-7, Iris-27 or Iris-42, where it can be stated that the patient will never die from cancer.

On the case card is recorded—

Father died at the age of 65 years from cancer of the oesophagus. During childhood the patient developed diphtheria as well as twice contracting measles.

There had been stomach symptoms over the past ten years. Radiographic examination two years previously had established nothing beyond a condition of insufficient gastric acidity. Radiographs taken eight days previously showed abnormality of the pylorus, delayed gastric function and inflammation of the large intestine.

Iris-15   **Male: 30 years—right iris**

At 38′ in the stomach zone (first minor zone), close examination shows a slight increase of whiteness which extends as a point into the intestinal ring. Indeed, the sign has a larger extent than this white point indicates and is more or less surrounded by interrupted arc-lines which begin at the pupillary margin at 34′ and 41′ and combine as a peak at the outer border of the intestinal zone (iris-wreath). (A) Since the white pointed sign lies within the larger sign, it indicates an inflammatory lesion of the pylorus which extends to the duodenum. However, the white point deviates upwards and suggests that the pylorus is displaced. This displacement arises as the result of pressure from a tumour exerted from below and behind against the pyloric section of the stomach.

Now observe the dark spot at 40′ immediately outside the iris-wreath and note the intensely white area immediately surrounding the spot in the third minor zone, indicating the cause of the duodenal condition. Also note the round, half-light and half-dark sign appearing immediately outside the iris-wreath at 22′ and which displaces the wreath circle towards the pupil (B). Medial to this sign, the intestinal zone shows a slackening of the fibres extending as a peak to the pupillary margin. Here also the stomach ring is smaller and narrower than in the remaining quadrants, indicating that the stomach is also displaced.

In the area outside the iris-wreath between the round sign and the iris-margin, a loosening of the iris fibres in the blood and muscle zones is to be seen (B). This also relates to the tumour, and indicates that as with the tissues of the stomach and duodenum, that of the pancreas is also involved. Similarly, the signs in the intestinal zone at 50' show the involvement of the intestine. This iris gives a positive indication for the onset of cancer of the pancreas. However, many years may pass before the condition is clinically diagnosable. The patient feels quite well apart from the repeated appearance of mild complaints. The case was followed for 10 years, when the cancer resulted in closure of the gall-duct and jaundice appeared. On surgical operation, the diagnosis of pancreatic cancer was confirmed.

Case record: The patient is a manual worker, 30 years old, single. Of the five brothers and sisters, three died as children. The parents are both still alive and healthy. The complaints at the first consultation were: stomach pains, eructations and back pains. The patient was symptom-free after the fifth treatment.

An iris with a fine compact structure always signifies a sensitive nervous system. On considering such an iris, it should be remembered that the patient feels everything much more acutely than the person showing an iris with a coarse structure of the tissue fibres.

The white cloud-like concentrations show a tendency to rheumatic pains, but since there is also continuity out to the iris-rim, there will be no marked encumbrance. The nerve rings (= contraction rings) reflect a general disturbance in calcium metabolism. In such irides every smallest sign should be noted, especially in those areas where the nerve rings show interruption. In the sector 10-20', the absence of lineal continuity in the nerve rings shows that there are disturbances in the organs projected in those areas: mouth, neck and back.

At 11' and 13', small dark points are to be seen in the fifth minor zone, indicating involvement of the throat. Small dark signs at the iris-rim (C) relate to the thyroid and parathyroid glands. These glands regulate calcium metabolism. In the area 16-18', several small dark signs extend outwards from the iris-wreath to the sixth minor zone, showing disturbances affecting the thoracic vertebrae (D). At 16-17' in the fifth minor zone and at 19-20' in the fourth minor zone, there are signs of tumour formation. At these locations the fine white lines appear to be pushed apart in arc formation and are not to be confused with lacunae. The sign at 19-20' lies in the area for lumbar vertebrae. From 20', a segment of nerve ring extends in a straight line to 27'. The straight course of the line is also of significance and is the subject for later research.

From 27' to 29' the nerve ring is again interrupted. In this sector, two thick white zig-zag radials are to be seen extending from the iris-wreath to the iris-rim, indicating the presence of painful conditions. The long dark sign with small black signs at 28', adjacent to the iris-wreath, shows involvement of the right kidney and a suspicion of kidney stones. A patient showing such signs will experience pain in the loin. (E)

From 30-36', two nerve rings may be seen with a short interruption at 34' originating from the dark sign which commences at the iris-wreath (F). This represents a suprarenal condition. Between 36' and 43' the nerve rings are frequently interrupted, suggesting the existence of conditions affecting stomach, duodenum, pancreas, liver and gall-bladder, and diaphragm.

From the above references, it will be evident that the nerve ring interruptions indicate those areas where disturbances exist. The zones in which they appear should also be noted as suggesting which tissue e.g. vascular, muscular, osseous, etc., is involved.

In general, there is a disturbance of calcium metabolism involving the parathyroid glands as principal regulators and producing various symptoms of a cramp-like nature, e.g. calf-cramps in the legs.

Iris-16   **Female: 27 years—right iris**

On first examination of the gastro-intestinal zone the sign at 38-45', which has the appearance of an obliquely suspended lacuna, is immediately apparent. The sign begins at the pupillary margin at 43-45' and indicates that there is a marked laxity of the tissues of the duodenum. The functional and structural damage resulting from it is indicated by the dark to black streaks within the lacuna. Likewise, the oblique white line within the sign suggests the presence of adhesions (A).

A state of faulty nutrition may be deduced from the peaked dilatations of the whole of the iris-wreath. The four small black points at 37-38' in the second major zone are signs for disease of the pancreas. However, the principal indication for the pancreas is shown by the black rhomboid sign at 22' in the second major zone. This sign indicates that the pathology is sealed off and as with the other signs described, is not giving rise to any prominent symptoms (B).

The black sign at 38-39' in the second and third major zones is a biliary sign. Since there are no white lines arising from the pupil to traverse the area, then no prominently painful conditions are present. The sign indicates biliary stasis, secondary to the adhesions affecting the duodenum and giving rise to gallstones (C).

The diagnosis is: duodenal pathology (duodenitis) resulting in insufficient discharge of bile and pancreatic secretion into the intestine, with consequent disturbance of the whole intestinal function. The symptoms are: intestinal colic with a tendency to diarrhoea. Since the signs are so strongly expressed in the right iris, they may be regarded as suggesting an inherited predisposition.

The brown fleck at 41' in the first major zone near to the margin of the pupil (below the light reflex) indicates the presence of a toxin deposit. When such a deposit is found at the principal focus of any disease condition, it indicates that the prognosis is poor and that cancerous changes may develop.

On the case record is noted: The patient is a hairdresser, 27 years of age and single. The father is 53 years of age and suffers from rheumatism. The mother died from thrombosis at the age of 43 years. Of the seven brothers and sisters of the mother, almost all died at about the age of 50 years, of which one had cancer and another thrombosis. The patient complained of belching and severe flatulence with attacks of colic from time to time. There was alternating diarrhoea and constipation.

The kidney area shows a large long closed lacuna at 28', indicating a previous condition now resolved. However, since the sign extends so far towards the outer iris-rim, the possibility of ptosis should be considered. The sign at 31' shows involvement of the suprarenal body (D). The assumption of renal ptosis is confirmed by the presence of inflammatory adhesions affecting the duodenum and extending throughout the abdominal cavity as far as the groin, as shown by the numerous fine transversals.

The intensely white colouring and the large dark lacunae and dark scurf-rim between 30' and 50' is particularly noticeable.

Consider the group of large lacunae at 43-50′ in the second and third major zones (E), showing a basic weakness of the respiratory organs: lungs and bronchi. Diametrically opposite, at 12′ in the area for throat, a lacuna indicates weakness of the air-passages (F). In the presence of such signs, one can safely assume either that the ancestors suffered from asthma, or that the patient has a history of whooping cough. Opposite to the dark scurf-rim, which is widest between 40′ and 50′, dense white deposits are to be seen at 8-17′ in the sixth minor zone. Whereas the dark scurf-rim indicates suppressed elimination from insufficient activity of the skin, the dense white deposits show encumbrance of the sinuses and mucous membranes of the naso-pharynx.

The small lacuna at 7′, close to the iris-wreath, which is still open, and the large closed lacuna at 5′ in the third to fifth minor zones, are signs for laxity affecting the frontal region and the forepart of the cranium (G).

Diametrically opposite to the lacuna at 5′, there is a large dark sign at 35′ in the third to fifth minor zones (H). This long sign, enclosing small black signs, shows a chronic condition of the caecum involving the peritoneum. This sign should not be regarded as a lacuna, but as suggesting pathology affecting the peritoneum, colon and appendix, with adherence and dehydration of the tissues, as shown by the white cross-lines. The adhesions will have involved the ureter and ovarian tube. The large lacuna in the kidney area has probably arisen from the same background, in which tissue weakness and suppurative conditions arise from urinary stasis.

The fact that the iris-wreath, hence the first major zone, is displaced downwards and not upwards, indicates that there is a displacement within the abdominal cavity but that it does not arise from a tumour. In this case, the displacement involves the kidney (large kidney sign at 28′), suprarenal bodies (two small lacunae at 31′ and 33′) and the gall-bladder (dark sign at 37-38′).

The transversals seen at 30-35′ in the third major zone show the presence of adhesions within the pelvis and extending up to the caecum (J). Where thin white cross-lines extend from the caecal area to the leg area, it is often found that a gravitation abscess may be present. Years may pass in such cases before outward drainage is established. Meanwhile, the patient is progressively afflicted by pains, together with shivering and variable febrile reactions. Intense sciatic pain and even acute or chronic rheumatism may often appear. However, if the abscess opens then the symptoms are relieved.

The small black sign with fine white transversals seen at 25′ in the sixth minor zone (K) is suggestive of tissue destruction (abscess) and should be related to the comments made above. This sign lies in the area for vagina and since the white lines radiate as far as the iris-rim then irritation and burning sensations within the vagina and at the orifice are indicated.

Iris-17   **Male: 42 years—right iris**

The first major zone has no prominent white border and there are no markedly white radiations over the second major zone. This signifies that the patient does not suffer intense pain. In such persons the pain of any disease process is never violent, and indeed, the coarse texture of the iris suggests that the patient can endure a great deal but that disease conditions generally fail to resolve completely. In his view, he has no time for that.

The first minor zone shows many black radiating streaks, of which some are short and some long, showing a chronic state of the gastric mucosa with involvement of the muscle layer. These signs indicate a tendency to degeneration of the mucous membrane with formation of ulcers. From 15′ to 45′ the black streaks are strongly marked and extend over the widened second minor zone and even beyond into the third minor zone.

At 30-50′ the first minor zone is much wider and suggests that the stomach is displaced downwards and to the right. In this connection note the signs in the gastro-intestinal ring at 40-44′. Of the three dark lacunae here lying one under the other, the uppermost and largest begins at the pupil, whereas the third and smallest lies outside the intestinal zone (iris-wreath) (A). Since the uppermost of the signs commences at the pupillary margin, then participation of the central nervous system is implied. The lowest lacuna lies outside the iris-wreath (sympathetic N.S) and adjacent to it a markedly darkened area is seen obliquely below extending into the third major zone as far as the liver area. The area is covered by large white flakes, indicating catarrhal inflammation with consequent swelling of the liver. This condition would press the pylorus and duodenum downwards, thus explaining the state of ptosis suggested by the widened stomach zone.

The signs shown at 36-43' indicate adhesions arising from ulcerous processes affecting pylorus and duodenum. These are the four dark streaks which radiate from the pupil and extend into the second minor zone. Adjacent to the iris-wreath in the third minor zone, two small elongated black signs indicate the presence of further adhesions. The white wisp sign leading to the liver area suggests inflammation (B).

Interpretation of these signs would usually include symptoms of intense pain, but that is not the case here. The patient, a beer distributor, small, corpulent and with abdominal ptosis, carried on his business every day, and since he himself was a driver, also had to perform physical work. When one day a severe gastric haemorrhage occurred and I was consulted, the patient explained that he had never had stomach symptoms and declined to believe that there was a gastric ulcer present. X-ray examination confirmed a condition of pyloric ulcer. In this case there must have been a condition of paralysis of the sensory nervous elements, as suggested by the three lacunae lying obliquely one under the other.

The large long closed lacuna at 35', which extends from the iris-wreath to the sixth minor zone, suggests that some chronic disease process within the abdominal cavity affecting the caecum has existed for a long time, perhaps even from youth, but has now been resolved. Since this lacuna also displaces the iris-wreath inwards, then there is also participation of the vegetative nervous system. The white border surrounding the sign is also projected to the pupillary margin, suggesting that the central nervous system is also being influenced. The short transversal seen at the iris-rim shows the presence of adhesions following operation or injury (C).

Apart from this large lacuna, the iris is covered with elongated small lacunae, together with large, wide and open lacunae. The signs generally are not so sharply defined as those seen in the preceding illustration (Iris-16) and the looseness of the structure gives the whole iris a grey colour. This looseness is not a favourable sign, especially in view of the sign formation in the areas for stomach and duodenum, which is so striking. In this connection, the flattening of the iris-rim at 33-43' should be noted, which with the gastro-duodenal signs suggests a pre-cancerous condition. The white clouds in the sixth minor zone, which extend to the iris-rim, are also prominent.

The small white clouds, seen immediately outside the iris-wreath between the dark lacunae, are signs found in rheumatic conditions and show inflammation of the tissues. If the signs are still very white, an acute phase is indicated, but if they become more greyish, then the acute phase has resolved. If the signs develop a yellow to brown colour, a late stage of gout is suggested.

The bright white cloud, seen at 50′ in the third major zone, implies severely painful conditions affecting the right shoulder. A similar large bright white cloud at 38′ in the third major zone (liver) suggests pain arising from an inflammatory process (D).

In this case, where no dark scurf-rim is to be seen at the outer edge of the iris, a good elimination through the skin is available. The patient drinks and sweats a great deal, but although he takes plenty of nourishment, the general health is not of the best, as shown by the lacunae in the ciliary zone. That is due to the organs in the gastro-intestinal zone, in which pathological disturbances arise from faulty nutrition.

Considering the large elongated sign at 29′, which reaches to the pupillary margin, and noting the diametrically opposite sign at 60′, which is also elongated, in relation to it (E), it may be stated that there is a condition of disharmony present ("The head desires otherwise than the feet"). Such patients come for treatment only when it is too late, whereas the patient represented by Iris-16 attends much sooner for treatment on account of the pains which arise as a consequence of his more sensitive nervous system (fine white nerve lines in the iris).

Eight years after the first gastric haemorrhage the patient died from a sudden violent haemorrhage. Diagnosis: carcinoma of the stomach.

Iris-18   **Female: 57 years—right iris**

The first minor zone is seen as a bright ring around the pupil. The area from 13′ to 17′ is perhaps somewhat lighter in shade. A very white stomach ring is generally suggestive of an inflammatory condition of the mucous membrane, and since the white signs also appear at the outer demarcation of the stomach zone, a rheumatic condition of the muscle layer is also implied.

At 42′ in the first minor zone a wedge-shaped sign is seen commencing at the outer edge of the stomach area, which has a heavy white border and a black centre. Following the white bordering lines outwards it is seen that the black centre continues as a long black line through the intestinal zone, beyond which the white lines continue outwards to the iris-rim. The white iris-wreath in this section is also thickened, from which white lines radiate outwards into the blood zone (A).

The direction of the white wedge-sign inwards towards the stomach zone may be regarded as implying some outside cause. The white zigzag lines which extend to the iris-rim show the presence of painful conditions and since the area 42-43′ in the ciliary zone corresponds to the arm, then painful symptoms affecting the limb are to be expected. The white cloud seen covering the third major zone at 50′ suggests that the shoulder is also implicated in these painful conditions.

Considering the area diametrically opposite at 12-13′ (mouth), the similarity of indications suggests the possibility of a connection. The hand-mouth line is the nutrition line, hence the digestive weakness suggested by the downward displacement of the gastro-intestinal zone may refer back to faulty nutrition. Since these signs appear so strikingly in the right iris, a hereditary predisposition can be assumed.

Referring now to the signs which extend from 32′ to 39′, it is seen that the white lines which demarcate the sign commence wide apart at the pupillary margin and run down to join together at the iris-wreath (37′). The stomach zone in this area is narrower than in the remaining circle. Careful examination shows a dark to black longish point at 37′ in the stomach zone which has some connection with the black sign in the intestinal zone. The signs lying within the peaked angle formed by the two oblique white lines (transversals) must be interpeted together. The upper white transversal begins at 41′ in the first minor zone and proceeds in an arc to the iris-wreath at 37′. The line then continues running obliquely to meet the iris-rim at 36′. The lower white transversal begins at the point where the upper branch crosses the iris-wreath and extends in a straight line back to the stomach ring at 35′. Since the white demarcating lines (the two transversals) run obliquely to the normal radial course of the iris fibres, then it may be taken that extensive adhesions and agglutinations have developed secondary to ulcerous processes and that the duodenum and pylorus are involved (B).

Diametrically opposite to the narrowed section of the stomach ring, a widened section of the bright stomach zone is seen, which represents the anterior wall of the stomach. This sign indicates that the stomach has dropped (gastroptosis) and that a strain has been set up at the level of the duodenum, since the suspending ligaments prevent the duodenum from following the course of the stomach. Thus, the conditions arising from the adhesions are aggravated still more.

Referring to the large subdivided black sign at 35-40′ below the signs already discussed (C), this sign lies outside the iris-wreath in the third and fourth minor zones and should be regarded as a pancreas sign.

Consider the dark sign at 3′ in the first minor zone, in which there are two small elongated black signs, a larger sign and a quite small point (D). This sign suggests that there must have been a large gastric ulcer affecting the anterior wall of the stomach and which healed with considerable scar tissue formation. Diametrically opposite to this sign at 31′, there is a large dark sign in the first minor zone which extends as a peak to the iris-wreath (E). At this location (as also at 3′) there is the cross-over from the anterior to the posterior wall of the stomach (lesser curvature). It would seem that the ulcer affecting the anterior wall has formed cicatrices which extend as far as the lesser curvature. This conclusion is supported by the white constriction sign observed at 4-5′ in the stomach zone. It may be assumed that the condition is due to trauma from a blow, since the sign is bordered by oblique white lines (transversals).

The sign at 32′ in the first major zone is also to be considered in this connection. Here an oblique thick white line extends outwards through the iris-wreath into a large white cloud demarcated by white arc-lines, which extend as far as the fifth minor zone (bone zone) to form a half-white, half-black lacuna (F). This sign refers to the kidney. The white cloud signifies inflammation, the arc-lines—dilatation, and the long black signs lying one under the other—loss of organ substance. Since the lowermost of the black signs is wider than it is long, it is to be presumed that there was an abscess of the kidney at some time. The sign as a whole indicates displacement of the organ in the abdominal cavity (floating kidney). The increased whitening at 40-43′ and 46-48′ outside the iris-wreath should be mentioned in this connection. One assumes that the inflamed kidney is lying close to the duodenum and large intestine and that these organs, together with the surrounding tissues, are involved in the pathology.

In this context, the thin white transversal extending as an arc from 43′ to 48′ in the second minor zone, and the two arc-lines which begin at the iris-wreath at 44′ and 48′ to form a peak in the first minor zone, must also be considered (G). These arc-lines, as also the inward deviation of the iris-wreath at 39-43′ and 45-48′, indicate pressure from without, i.e. from the displaced and enlarged kidney. The narrowing of the stomach ring at 32-40′ similarly indicates participation. Tracing the ultimate end of the arc-line at 31′, it is seen that this runs obliquely to the normal course of the iris-fibres, thus suggesting that the kidney condition has arisen from outside influences.

The case record reads as follows: the patient is 57 years of age. Weight 57 kg. Height 1.62 m. Married with two children. The patient's father died at the age of 52 years from a tumour below the stomach and her mother died at the age of 81 years from senile decay. A sister of the father died between 50 and 60 years of age from tuberculosis and the grandmother on the mother's side died at the age of 50 years from tuberculosis.

During childhood the patient suffered frequent attacks of pain which began in the feet and worked up to the head. The last attack of this kind ended with loss of consciousness and the coughing of blood. At the age of 47 years, abdominal pains appeared for the first time, beginning under the ribs on the right side. The pains were cramplike, short but violent, and recurred within a year. For the past year the pains had occurred every fourteen days, especially appearing after exertion and lasting for some hours, but less violent than before. They reduced on resting. During the last few months the patient had spent most of the time in bed. Defaecation was not possible without the use of purgatives. The attending physician did not know how to begin with the patient. He had probably said that there might be a tumour lying below the stomach and that if the trouble did not improve, an operation would be necessary. On the basis of irisdiagnosis, I treated the patient for a condition of floating kidney, with the result that she put on weight and the pains disappeared.

Six months later the crampy pains re-appeared following an accident. When these pains subsided, the patient then complained of pain in the right hip and leg, when Lasegue's sign was found to be positive. After a further two years the patient again presented herself complaining of giddiness, but explained that she had been able to work for the whole of the previous summer without complaint. The weight was now 62 kg.

Another example: Shortly after this episode a patient consulted me showing the same large kidney sign. The sign was also displaced to the left, but with the difference that the whole sign was dark and not as in the above case where the one half appeared white. There were the same arc-lines in the kidney area, as well as arc-lines in the first and second minor zones at 45-48'. The lack of white signs denoting inflammation explains why no pains were present in this case.

I still remembered the first consultation of about five to six years before. At that time I told the patient after the iris examination that he had a floating kidney and that the kidney must be lying somewhat forward in the abdominal cavity. He was quite astonished and then told me that after lengthy investigations the same diagnosis had been made. He had been treated already for all possible diseases on account of a tumour lying anteriorly just below the surface of the abdominal wall, and that even following a uroscopy the condition had not been clarified. The cause of the condition was a fall from a scaffold. The symptoms, which had appeared only a long time after the fall, were colicky and violent. However, there had been no more symptoms for some years.

To return to iris-18: In addition to the signs already described, it remains to elucidate the subdivided sign appearing at 16-18' in the second major zone (H). The small lacunae lying one under the other, containing fine white lines running across the signs, suggest that a shrivelling of the tissues has taken place. This development is probably a secondary consequence of the floating kidney and the general dropping of the abdominal organs.

This abdominal ptosis produces a considerable back strain. To this is added the displacement produced by the detached kidney. In addition, the sign at 20' in the second major zone indicates swelling. It is a longish dark sign, subdivided into three parts, and surrounded by a white border (J). Adjacent to it at 21' there is a white transversal. If the back strain increases it produces a sign similar to the subdivided lacuna.

Opposite to this sign at 50', a large white area is seen in the third major zone, indicating an inflammatory condition of the shoulder. This condition goes with the back strain. The sign formation at 52' in the second and third major zones suggests that there are disturbances of the neck which would be helped by vertebral adjustment of the neck and back. The uniform course of the iris-fibres in the second and third major zones otherwise indicates no serious disturbance.

Iris-19   **Male: 18 years—right iris**

On close examination of the pupil, an outward displacement of the pupillary margin is seen covering the segment 13-17', where it appears as though a long rectangular piece has been cut out. This suggests a severe disturbance involving the pylorus which could easily lead to the development of ulceration. On further observation of the iris fibres at 10-12' in the first and second minor zones, a sign with its point towards the pupil is seen covering both zones, and indicates the existence of adhesions affecting the anterior wall of the stomach (A). These individual signs will be further discussed in detail.

Considering first the gastro-intestinal zone, a large sign arising from the pupillary margin is seen at 40'. This sign lies within the iris-wreath and on close observation is seen to include three small black signs, in addition to the larger long black sign (B). Immediately below this location, two white parallel lines run from the pupillary margin to the iris-rim, enclosing a small long and point-like sign (C). These signs together constitute a connected group and indicate severe cicatrisation of the duodenum and pylorus. The presence of the white wavy lines running outwards suggests the presence of severe pains.

Below this group of signs is a long rectangular sign which sits on the large lacuna like a cap. The rectangular sign and the closed lacuna lie outside the second minor zone (iris-wreath) and are to be considered as relating to the head of the pancreas (D). The rectangular sign on top indicates adhesions between pancreas and duodenum. That not merely the pylorus and the lower part of the duodenum are affected by adhesions to the surrounding tissues is shown by the large sign in the second minor zone which is subdivided into four sections and has been displaced somewhat by the large lacuna (E). This sign shows adhesions affecting the descending part of the duodenum. These conditions affect the discharge of secretion from the pancreas, and the large lacuna representing the head of the organ has probably developed as a consequence. The intense white clouds immediately below indicate the presence of inflammation. The small black points at 38′ in the third major zone, with their dense borders, suggest the probability of gallstones and a gallbladder affected pathologically by inflammatory changes.

But the young man's illness is not limited to these conditions. On considering the gastro-intestinal zone at 17-20′, it is seen that the iris fibres in this area continue into the second major zone and that the border (iris-wreath) cannot be identified. This suggests that there are adhesions connecting the posterior wall of the stomach with the pancreas and duodenum. The presence of inflammatory conditions is also shown by the intense whiteness in the area. Pains arising from between the shoulder blades are indicated by the white wavy lines which radiate outwards to the iris-rim.

At 48-53′ in the second minor zone several dark to black signs are seen which take the form of two peaks pointing outwards and with one open and two closed lacunae adjacent to them on the outside of the iris-wreath (F). These are signs for adhesions affecting the large intestine and are to be considered in relation to those in the duodenal area.

A marked constriction of the colon with inflammation is suggested by the white sign at 57′, where the inwardly directed peak almost reaches the pupil (G). The intensely white radiating fibres in the segment 50-10′ indicate the presence of headaches.

The caecal area should also be mentioned. An outwardly directed intestinal peak at 33′ is flanked by two closed lacunae in the third minor zone (H). This sign grouping indicates the existence of a suppurative appendix with massive adhesions and abscess formation affecting the surrounding tissues. The abscess formation is shown by the small rhomboid-like signs with their thick white borders in the fourth minor zone. Similar signs are seen below the large lacuna at 37′.

The course of the symptoms in this patient will provide better understanding of the disease condition: After the 18 year old patient had been attended by many doctors with no improvement, the parents brought him to me. The previous history included the following symptoms: from birth there had been vomiting,

68

diarrhoea and feverish conditions with variable intermissions. There was inflammation and swelling of the glands in the groins after exertion, especially from long walks and gymnastics.

After examination and explanation to the mother, it was suggested that the boy be taken out of school for a period of three months, so that he could be cared for at home, enabling proper attention to be given to diet and punctual medication. A good result was recorded at the end of the period.

The parents now considered that the boy should return to school. The advice to postpone resumption for a further three months was not accepted and the boy's condition soon deteriorated. On being called up for military service the patient was directed into hospital where a good internist took charge of him. After detailed examinations over six months, during which time tuberculosis and other possibilities were investigated, the existence of gastro-intestinal ulcerations was established and a condition of chronic pancreatitis was treated. Belladonal and Pancreon were prescribed. The preparation Pancreon was first included after the patient had explained to the doctor that he had improved so well on my prescription of the Pancreon preparation. After the patient had somewhat recovered in two years of hospitalisation and rest, he had to enlist as a soldier, but was able to undertake manual work during his voluntary time in the business conducted by his father and is now able to continue with slight interruption.

On comparing the structure of the iris fibres with that shown in Iris-18, the laxity of the structure is immediately obvious. This laxity ('combed-hair') gives a generally grey colour to the iris and is a sign for premature aging. The whole ciliary zone, including blood, muscle and bone zones, participate in this state.

Note that the thick wavy lines extend as far as the iris-rim without the formation of clouds in the sixth minor zone. This indicates good elimination through the skin with resolution of the inflammation by profuse perspiration. However, the heavy sweating can be dangerous if insufficient liquid is taken and no regard is paid to the sodium chloride level of the blood. A salt deficiency quickly arises when too much is lost in perspiration. Only in this way can water be eliminated. However, watery stools can occur from inability of the intestinal wall to reabsorb water because of sodium chloride shortage. A further consequence is insufficient absorption of nutrients from the chyme.

Disturbance of the kidney is to be seen from the large dark sign at 29' in the second major zone (J). This sign widens as far as 31' and also extends too far towards the iris border, indicating a swelling and displacement of the organ and probably attributable to the adhesions affecting the ureters in the pelvis. The long black sign at 26', together with the large dark area at 21-24' suggests considerable weakness of the bladder and genital organs (K).

The large dark sign extending from the iris-wreath almost to the iris-margin, widening outwards across the area 1-4', corresponds to the position for the pituitary gland (L). When large signs like this are seen in the area for anterior cerebrum to indicate pituitary conditions, then developmental deficiency of the glands of internal secretion is to be expected.

Iris-20   **Male: 23 years—right iris**

In general, the stomach ring covers the whole of the first major zone. Therefore, the stomach zone is too large relative to the intestinal zone and implies the probability of enlargement of the stomach.

Very many black signs are to be found in the stomach area originating at the pupillary margin, some of which cross over the stomach ring. These signs indicate deterioration of the gastric mucous membrane. When such black signs are present with a stomach ring which is otherwise too white, then the existence of severe heartburn reaching up into the throat may be assumed. From the intense black signs at 17', 25', 34' and 35', particular implication of the posterior wall of the stomach is indicated.

The black wedge-sign at 41' with its peak directed towards the intestinal zone, below which a white sign is seen, signifies the cicatrisation of the pylorus from inflammatory conditions. That severe pains are present is shown by the white lines which radiate outwards from the wedge sign to extend to the iris-rim (A).

At 39-42' the iris-wreath takes the form of a straight line composed of a succession of white points. Immediately below at 38' a dark line is to be seen which commences at the pupil and breaking through the wreath line extends outwards as far as the fourth minor zone. A similar dark line is seen at 35'. This sign originates in the area for the caecum, whereas the former line breaks through the wreath in the area for the duodenum. In association with these signs note the large transversal which begins at 39′ in the fifth minor zone and ends at 35′ at the iris-rim. At this point another small transversal is seen which crosses the larger (B).

From these signs it may be assumed that an abdominal injury has been sustained, resulting in tissue damage affecting the caecum and duodenum. Whether the gall-bladder and liver were also affected cannot be definitely asserted. However, the round dark sign enclosing black points seen at 38′ in the fifth minor zone indicates that the gall-bladder is now involved (gall-bladder inflammation, biliary stasis, gall-stones).

The large closed lacuna at 35-38′ in the third and fourth minor zones indicates that the pancreas has been affected by the stasis of its secretion. The presence of white clouds also suggests the presence of inflammation (C).

Diagnosis: Chronic gastritis with ulceration, inflammation of the duodenum, gall-bladder and pancreas with adhesions.

The following are the most important phases of the history:
1930—a severe blow was sustained affecting the right side close to the stomach. The attending physician diagnosed slight bruising of the pleura and prescribed a local salve. Since the complaints were no better after a year and meanwhile appeared very severe, the patient came under my care. My findings were: inflammation and adhesions affecting stomach, intestine and liver areas together with involvement of the right kidney. I accordingly advised reference to a specialist for the purpose of radiographic examination and possible operation, but the specialist concerned laughed the patient out when he heard my diagnosis.

After lengthy but unsuccessful treatment from different physicians, the patient was in hospital for one week during 1935 where the usual stomach and gall-bladder examinations were carried out together with a uroscopy, with the result that he was discharged as a malingerer. The doctor consulted a short time after diagnosed irritation of the appendix and referred the patient to another hospital, where a duodenal ulcer was confirmed and treatment instituted. The pains were probably eased for a time but soon afterwards re-appeared unbearably severe.

The patient then went to a specialist for internal diseases, who diagnosed gastro-intestinal catarrh with inflammation of the gall-bladder. After a long period of incapacity for work he was referred to hospital by the company doctor for observation and was treated for catarrh of the stomach and intestines. Subsequently, he was called up for military exercise, but after a short time the pains were again very severe and he was discharged. The specialist now sent him into hospital for surgery. The condition found was: adhesions of gall-bladder, duodenum and stomach.

The patient again attended for consultation in January 1938 to complain of similar pains. He was alternatively capable of work for a fortnight and ill for a fortnight. This continued until the end of 1938 when light work was suggested. Until that time he had to work the whole day as a plumber in a stooping position.

On considering the ciliary zones generally, it will be seen that there is a similar degree of laxity of the iris-stroma as with Iris-19. The existence of small closed and open lacunae between 13′ and 50′ make the blood, muscle and bone zones appear dark. This alone immediately suggests a condition of anaemia affecting these tissues. Viewed correctly, the iris shows a protrusion of the first major zone with a sunken condition of the third, fourth and fifth minor zones. The plane of the sixth minor zone is again forwards. According to French researchers in iridology, this is also a sign for a severe degree of anaemia. It also indicates considerable weakness of the organs and tissues represented in the blood, muscle and bone areas.

Diametrically opposite to the large dark segments in the pulmonary and thoracic areas (42-50′) a similar dark area is seen representing the dorsum (D). The most prominent sign lies in the segment showing the profile aspect and consequently indicates that there is a most severe degree of exhaustion which is not easy to influence. A similar consideration also applies to the white deposits seen at 33-42′, referring to disturbances in the abdominal cavity which are of a more difficult nature (profile aspect).

The closed lacuna at 23′ in the second major zone shows that the bladder has been affected by an inflammatory condition (E). Similarly, the closed lacuna at 28′ suggests a resolved inflammation of the renal pelvis (F). The intensely white radials from the iris-wreath indicate inflammatory stimulation of the tissues.

In this case, rapid elimination of toxic matter through the skin is not possible as was the case with Iris-19. This is to be seen from the presence of white cloud formations in the sixth minor zone and although the patient perspires heavily, there is insufficient elimination as against the considerable absorption of toxic material from the bowel.

The large open lacunae between 42′ and 50′ are of particular interest. At 43-45′ long wavy white radials are seen showing chronic bronchial catarrh (G). These radials are diametrically opposite the peak of the dark lacuna seen at 12-16′, representing a condition of chronic catarrh of the pharynx (H).

The small black point-like signs between 10′ and 16′ in the third major zone suggest that there is focal infection of the teeth and that the tonsils are encumbered. In view of the conditions present in the abdominal cavity, especially the chronic inflammatory conditions focussed on the appendix, it would indeed be remarkable if the tonsils were not diseased, or that the teeth should remain healthy in the presence of general exhaustion.

The large dark area between 43′ and 50′ shows a general weakness of the lung tissue. When this is seen to be so prominent in the right iris, it suggests that tubercular conditions must have existed along the ancestral line. There was a history of asthma in the ancestors and the patient himself suffered severe whooping cough. If a lacuna is also seen in the heart area of the left iris, then the development of an asthmatic syndrome in old age may be assumed, if tuberculosis or even cancer does not terminate life before.

In my view, an ideal medical science would need to include not only the treatment of the suffering patient, but also recognition of the latent tendency to specific diseases and so prevent their development. In this respect, irisdiagnosis provides the only means which can show the pathological trends and insidious processes.

The case record notes the following:
The patient was 25 years old, single, the sixth child of six siblings. The father suffers from haemorrhoids. The mother suffered at the age of 50 years from cerebral sclerosis and died at the age of 68 years from rectal cancer. The maternal grandparents both died from pneumonia.

The patient died from pulmonary tuberculosis at the age of 38 years.

At 40-45' there is a somewhat oblique complex of lines commencing at the pupillary margin and extending into the intestinal zone, indicating that pylorus and duodenum are affected by adhesions (A). The dark sign at 38' at the edge of the first major zone, which appears as though it originates from the pupillary margin is to be considered as a pancreas sign. It is not a part of the intestinal zone. There are adhesions of the pancreas with stomach and duodenum (B).

In relation to this, consider the uppermost white line beginning at 40' in the small white cloud immediately above the pancreas sign at the outer edge of the first major zone and extending in a large arc to the iris-rim at 34', together with the lowermost line which begins at 35' in the first major zone and ends at 33' at the iris-rim. These signs indicate that there are displacements in the abdominal cavity (C).

The narrowing of the intestinal ring between 30' and 39' is also an indication of displacement. In relation to this, note the many small transversals in the third major zone in the segment 30-40'. These signs indicate the presence of adhesions in the abdominal cavity. Such indications are found following peritoneal irritation or inflammation.

Also note the group of signs at 17-22' adjacent to the iris-wreath, where a thick white line forms an obtuse angle at the upper border, whereas the lower part of the complex cannot be identified as a white line but diffuses out gradually into normal iris structure (D). This sign complex should not be regarded as a lacuna, such as may be seen at 43-45' and 45-48' in the second major zone, but should be assessed as a subdivided defect-sign.

This shows damage to the pancreas, giving rise to chronically recurring back pain. Since the sign lies high, it shows that the pains are referred to the upper back between the shoulder blades.

In a patient found to have carcinoma of the pancreas, I have recently observed that where the signs were found in both irides, including the location at 23' left iris, pains simulating disease of the sigmoid flexure appeared in the abdomen. However, clinical and radiographic examination was negative. No evidence of cancer was detected. When the patient developed jaundice from obstruction of the gall-duct, he was submitted for surgical operation, which revealed: cancer of the pancreas.

Referring again to the signs at 17-22′, it is striking that the upper thick white line runs somewhat obliquely to the normal iris radial fibres. Subtended from this line are two other white lines at the middle and outer end, which also run obliquely to form two long signs of unequal size which are further subdivided (D). It is clear that the organ condition shown has arisen from injury to the back and involves adhesions between pancreas and stomach.

Comparing this with the previous iris, it is seen that in that case the signs are located at 35-45′ with the disturbances more in the right anterior upper abdominal region, whereas in the case of the present patient they appear in the back.

At the first consultation the patient complained of pains in the right abdomen extending from the groin to the gall-bladder, together with constipation and a boring pain in the back between the shoulder blades. Over a period of 14 days in a clinic, the patient had been examined and radiographed, but nothing was found. She was discharged with a direction to present herself again in six months time. There was only some nervousness present.

The two large dark lacunae between 42′ and 48′ in the second major zone (blood and muscle), which are immediately apparent, show the existence of a general weakness affecting the pulmonary system. (E) The lower of the two signs refers to the bronchi and the upper to the lung parenchyma. In this connection, since cardiac enlargement to the right produces stasis especially affecting the right lung, the condition of the heart should be considered. A detailed examination of the heart area in the left iris should be made to confirm cardiac involvement. In this case, the adhesions present in the abdominal cavity, and the condition of liver and pancreas resulting in a high position of the diaphragm, should be taken into consideration.

Also note the kidney sign at 28′. The structural formation of the sign suggests that the organ has become adherent to surrounding tissues as a result of an earlier disorder, this leading to stasis affecting the right side of the abdomen. (F)

The large signs to be seen at 9-15′ in the second and third major zones (G), diametrically opposite to the two large lacunae in the pulmonary areas, show the state of pharynx and trachea and should be partly assessed as lacunae. However, the small elongated black signs indicate tissue defects resulting from unresolved pharyngeal, tracheal and bronchial catarrh.

The white cloud at 45' in the third major zone (H), together with the scleral vascular signs, show that the condition is still unresolved. The small elongated dark sign at 23' in the fourth minor zone surrounded by a white border (J) shows the existence of catarrh of the bladder with present symptoms.

The generally fine structure of the iris fibres together with the white clouds and wisps indicate a basically rheumatic emphasis in this patient. With such a constitutional stress one should remember the tendency to focal infection and formation of stones. In relation to infective foci, note the small elongated signs visible at 35' in the second and third major zones (K). The white radial fibres in the fifth minor zone extending out to the iris-rim and the dark areas lying between show a tendency to nettlerash.

The white clouds at the outer edge of the iris between 25' and 29' indicate chronic inflammation and irritation of the vagina and surrounding organs, with burning sensations. These conditions are likely to have their origin in chronic catarrh of the uterus, as shown by the dark signs at 25-29' in the third major zone, which begin as a peak close to the iris-wreath. A transversal is seen at 25' and a black point is also visible at 22' within the dark angle, suggesting injury to the cervix and the possible formation of polypi (L).

The following notes appear on the case record:

The patient is a housewife, 43 years of age, married with two children. The father died from cancer of the liver at the age of 65 years, and the mother died from abdominal cancer at the age of 42 years. No information was given concerning other ancestors.

During childhood the patient contracted measles, scarlet fever and diphtheria. At 30 years of age she was twice operated upon for inguinal hernia, left and right. One year after the iris photograph was taken, the patient had a surgical operation on the uterus.

After 10 years, the patient again attended for consultation, complaining of pains in the chest, especially after swallowing solid food. Nothing special had been found on X-ray examination. The condition was again better after a short period of treatment.

The pupil is too small and shows an over-stimulated condition of the nervous system. The same conclusion is suggested by the compact iris structure in which the white radial lines appear as though tightly stretched.

The first major zone shows no obvious demarcation of the stomach ring and is on the whole too light in colour. This more intense colouring—not brilliant white as with inflammation—suggests the presence of severe burning sensations in the stomach. In spite of that, there can be a deficiency of stomach acid. Compare this with Iris-16 and Iris-18 and note that in the present case there is a lightening of the grey colour, whereas those illustrations show the intense white colour of inflammation.

On considering the relatively dark sign at 40' in the first major zone, it is seen that two black streaks radiate out from the pupil to cross the whole zone. Long black signs between white lines are also seen radiating out in the second major zone, which are a continuation of the signs in the gastro-intestinal zone. These black streaks and long signs are defect-signs, indicating that tissue has been damaged by inflammatory processes and scar-tissue adhesions have appeared. It should be noted that in this segment the white lines are not so straight as in the remainder of the iris (A).

This section from 22' to 28' in the first major zone also shows two longer and two shorter black lines. These signs are probably to be considered with those at 40' and show the implication of the posterior wall of the stomach, whereas the first sign relates to the pylorus and duodenum (B).

The black oval sign at 23-27' in the first and second major zones, which appears as though laid on, is a toxin deposit. Since this sign lies close to the black streaks, it confirms the severity of the stomach condition (B). The small black streak at 52', which radiates out from the second minor zone, together with the small black line within the peak of the intestinal dilatation at 7', are to be considered jointly as indicating adhesions affecting both large and small intestine (C).

From all these signs, bearing in mind their smallness and that the whole of the first major zone appears too small, it may be assumed that a cancerous condition has developed, accompanied by the onset of painful symptoms. An abnormal condition has already been confirmed by radiography.

At the first consultation the complaints were of stomach and abdominal pains, anal irritation and worms. The diagnosis was: adhesions affecting the posterior wall of the stomach. No worm signs are to be seen in the iris-picture. The signs discussed above are of a much more serious nature and have priority of importance. Since the treatment given, no further entries appear on the case record.

The striking appearance of radiating white lines in this iris probably arises from the strong contraction of the pupil. When such signs are present, particular attention should be given to the pupillary reaction to note whether an excessive degree of miosis exists which would affect the overall judgment of the condition. Stereoscopic examination of the iris would show that the first major zone is bulging forward while the second major zone is sunken. The former appearance signifies over-stimulation of the central and vegetative nervous systems, whereas the latter indicates weakness of the blood and muscle systems as in Iris-20.

The peripheral white clouds, which are particularly prominent between 10′ and 30′ (third major zone), show increased reactivity of the mucous membranes. In this case, there exists an increased resistance to the injurious materials taken up from the organs of the first major zone into the systems represented by the second major zone. The serious degree of involvement of the pulmonary system in the degenerative condition of the blood is expressed by the large dark segments at 42-45′ and 7-15′. However, since the overall darkening of the second major zone extends into the third major zone, there is already an encumbrance of the skeletal system. The bone marrow is thus no longer able to influence the blood condition in any favourable sense.

A short white transversal is seen at 30′ in the leg area which relates to the long black sign. These signs indicate damage to the leg probably resulting from an injury to the leg and foot (D).

The case record reads as follows: The patient is a land worker, 38 years of age, married with two children. The father is 68 years old and healthy, the mother is 64 years old and has been sickly for a long time. Of the five brothers and sisters to the father, one is small and one died from tuberculosis. The paternal grandfather died at the age of 50 years from tabes dorsalis after being confined to bed for ten years. The paternal grandmother suffered from gout and died from heart failure at the age of 65 years. The maternal grandfather suffered from haemoptysis in youth but has lived to the age of 70 years. The maternal grandmother died from senile weakness at the age of 89 years.

Iris-23   **Male: 29 years—right iris**

The size of the pupil is normal and it is evenly circular. The pupillary margin is too black and indicates a loss of functional capacity of the gastric mucous membrane. The gastro-intestinal zone is too small and suggests induration and poor assimilation. The outer border of the stomach ring is not visible.

The widening of the first major zone between 30' and 48' is to be taken as indicating ptosis of the abdominal organs generally. Between 37' and 43' a white line crosses the zone obliquely and at 43' there is a white wedge-sign containing a thin black streak. This sign complex has been produced by ulcerous processes affecting the duodenum. In this case it is probable that the stomach itself is not the origin of the condition (A).

The signs at 20-25' deserve special attention since they certainly suggest the greatest danger for the patient. The oblique zig-zag transversal beginning almost at the pupillary margin at 15' to run below almost vertically to the iris-wreath at 23', the small transversal outside the wreath in the third minor zone and the peaked black signs at 20' bordering the iris-wreath which interrupt the course of the white zig-zag transversal, taken together, certainly suggest a potential cancerous condition. Indeed, it is possibly already present. Ulcerous processes affecting the posterior wall of the stomach (lesser curvature) have been the origin of this condition (B).

The black lines radiating out from the pupillary margin at 51', 57', 3' and 6' to extend into the second major zone are signs for nervous exhaustion and indicate mento-emotional depletion and general lassitude. The white wavy lines seen in the second and third major zone appear somewhat strained and suggest the presence of severe pains affecting those locations where the white lines are clustered together and extend to the iris-rim.

The doctor in attendance had diagnosed a condition of duodenal ulcer. The patient had been variably treated by several doctors for gastric ulcers. On 21.3.39 he came under my care for haemorrhage of the stomach. After some initial improvement a haemorrhage again appeared on 28.4.39. With long intervals between, the patient remained under treatment until 1944 when he was called up for military service. Symptoms of gastric acidity, burning and retching were always present.

In this iris, a marked contraction of the iris-wreath with consequent restriction of the gastro-intestinal zone is seen in the kidney segment, with a dense white cloud and a dark sign below extending to the iris-rim (C). Such signs indicate chronic inflammation of the kidney involving tissue degeneration. The participation of the surrounding tissues (duodenum and large intestine) is shown by the dense white clouds in the area 40-50' adjacent to the iris-wreath.

Comparing this iris with the previous illustration, it will be noticed that the fibre structure appears less tense than is the case in Iris-22, probably due to the larger pupil. However, there is a more intense white colouring surrounding the first major zone of Iris-23 and there are no white flakes in the third major zone. Indeed, there are many small dark signs between the radiating white lines, which indicate that the blood system alone has to maintain resistance to the damaging materials absorbed from the gastro-intestinal tract, since the active resistance of the peripheral mucous membrane or of the lymphatic system is no longer available. In this case, elimination is transferred back to the intestines, with consequent reiteration of severe symptoms affecting these organs.

Even though Iris-22 shows severe disturbance of the nervous system, yet there is also a certain degree of apathy and loss of feeling in relation to the symptoms (asthenia). In the case of Iris-23, it is otherwise. Here, the conditions are expressed by repeated severe pains with unrest and general excitability.

As already stated, the contraction of the iris-wreath at 28', with the adjacent thick white cloud raises the question of renal pathology. The contraction of the wreath indicates an earlier inflammatory condition, while the thick white clouds show that the inflammation still persists. The small black points in this segment show loss of tissue integrity (defects). The presence of kidney stones will maintain the acute response.

From the black elongated signs in the fifth minor zone and the long dark sign at 29-30' in the leg area, it may be deduced that there is damage to the skeletal system and more especially to the bone marrow. (D)

Even though Iris-22 presents a severe condition of the stomach and intestine, with the possibility of malignant change, yet the pulmonary system encumbrance and the mucous membrane stress, to be assessed by the peripheral white flakes, inclines one rather to consider a likely tubercular degeneration, whereas Iris-23 suggests a disposition to induration and cancerous change.

Iris-24   **Female: 41 years—right iris**

The small white flakes seen in the first major zone portray inflammation of the gastric mucous membrane. The elongated black signs at 40', 31' and 25' in this zone are ulcer signs (A). These three signs deserve special mention, even though there are many other signs to indicate ulcerous processes, particularly between 45' and 50'.

The two elongated signs at 40' and 42', together with the black point at 29', are to be regarded as one sign-complex and represent ulcerous adhesions affecting the duodenum. Considerable involvement of the tissues behind and below must also exist. The wedge-sign at 30' is to be considered in the same context and indicates damage to the right kidney (B). Likewise with the signs at 40-50'.

Note that the whole of the first major zone is occupied by the stomach ring, except for the group of black signs at 47' which truly represents the intestine (C). Moreover, the gastro-intestinal zone in relation to the ciliary zones is too small and suggests a condition of poor assimilation, induration and malignancy.

Observe particularly the flattening of the pupillary ring between 35' and 50', and of the iris-rim at 33-43'. If this iris is compared with the next, then a condition of induration on a malignant basis may certainly be assumed. The narrowing of the stomach zone in the upper and lower quadrants is particularly apparent and is also to be seen in the next iris. These last signs described should be noted in the other iris illustrations.

The following notes appear on the case record: The patient is 41 years old and married with two children. The father is 69 years of age and healthy. The mother died at 68 years of age from cancer of stomach and liver. There was no information concerning other antecedents.

Comparing this iris with Iris-22, there are similar considerations with the exception of the nervous stress. In this case, the size of the pupil is normal and there are no tense white radials. However, the encumbrance affecting the respiratory organs is strongly evident, with prominent signs showing as dark areas and lacunae between 40' and 50' (D), and as the dark area at 10' with small black points in the segment 10-16' (E). Between 40' and 55' the small black points are situated in the second major zone, whereas those between 10' and 25' lie in the third major zone. Below these signs are many others which indicate tissue degeneration.

In accordance with the more recent research in histo-pathology, the origin of the iris signs may be explained as follows: When metabolic wastes collect in the tissue spaces the resultant deposits are without innervation and there is no immediate inflammatory reaction of the surrounding tissues. Therefore, no special iris-signs will appear during the early stage. However, with increased accumulation of deposited materials, pressure signs show as an elevation of the iris fibres. As pressure further increases to affect normally innervated tissues, an inflammatory response is initiated and the elevated iris-fibres acquire a white colouring (inflammation signs). Before this stage, there is almost nothing to be seen in the iris, if no attention is given to the slight elevation of the iris-fibres. Degeneration of the deposited material produces intoxication and destruction of the tissue-cells affected, so producing the black signs (defect signs) in the iris. The materials deposited will vary according to the nutritional intake and the nature of the degenerative change will determine whether cancer, tuberculosis or one of the other diseases will develop, showing a variable course and differential symptoms.

Comparing this iris with irides 22, 23 and 25, it will be seen from the white signs over the iris generally that the whole body is engaged in the struggle against auto-intoxication by increased reactivity (inflammatory reaction). In this case therefore, there is continued resistance of the lymphatic system, as is likewise indicated in Iris-22 by the white cloud formations in the third major zone. In both Iris-23 and Iris-25 the resistance of the lymphatic system is almost completely gone and especially in Iris-23, dark to black spaces have developed between the white radial lines.

From the existence of transversals at 15-20' in the second and third major zones of Iris-24, it may be deduced that adhesions of the pleura have resulted from an inflammatory reaction, a possible consequence of a tubercular condition. However, as already stated, cancer may develop where there is also a disposition to tuberculosis. Indeed, they may exist together. (F)

The physician in attendance detected a swelling below the right breast bone and thought that surgery would be necessary. At the first consultation the patient complained of epigastric pressure and heartburn. Stomach pains were relieved by eating. Defaecation was not possible without the aid of laxatives. The patient further complained of pain in the right thorax extending to the axilla. Eight years before, while suckling a child, a tumour had developed above the right mammary gland which did not afterwards recede. There was a nodule in the right breast the size of an egg.

The patient was referred to a clinic. Whether the cause for the present malignancy was the indurated tumour in the mammary gland or the earlier ulcerous processes affecting the stomach, was never ascertained. In any case, metastases were so extensive in the body that an operation on the breast or stomach was hopeless.

It might be assumed in such a condition as this that a special indication would appear in the iris. In all disease processes taking place in the body, the liver, as the most important and largest gland, inevitably participates in the disturbance as a detoxicating organ. This detoxication is achieved by the liver without its own tissues becoming affected, thus explaining the absence of any specific signs in the iris. A similar capacity is possessed by the spleen. Thus, in most cases where there is a severe degree of encumbrance, a darkening of the appropriate areas in the iris is seen (spleen: 20-25' left iris, liver: 35-40' right iris) in the third major zone. Only when damage occurs to the cells and tissues of the liver and spleen would other iris-signs appear in those areas. A particularly evident sign, where these organs are the subject of tissue-cell damage, is the prominent formation of conjunctival blood vessels adjacent to the organ areas.

The flattening of the iris-rim at 35-40', to be seen both in this iris and Iris-25, is a sign that pathological changes affecting the parenchymatous cells are taking place in the liver. Displacement of the iris-wreath towards the pupil in the same segment suggests enlargement of the liver and implication of the vegetative nervous system.

In Irides—20, 21 and 22, the special involvement of the pulmonary system has been described. Since the signs are so strongly expressed in the right iris, hereditary encumbrance is indicated. If additional signs are present showing previous severe bronchitis and whooping cough, the patient's attention should be directed to any bad breathing habits. The presence of signs in the kidney areas indicates the need to support renal capacity to eliminate toxic products through the kidneys and not merely to restrict the content of the diet.

Iris-25   **Male: 72 years—right iris**

In this case the gastro-intestinal zone is too small generally, as well as being even more contracted at 60-10′ and 22-45′. The displacements involved are caused by marked swelling of the liver.

The black signs in the stomach zone at 20′, 26′, 34′, 37′ and 52′ are defect-signs originating in ulcerous processes which have produced considerable cirrhosis. The white colour seen between the black streaks at 10-20′ and 35-50′ suggests that there is severe inflammation of the stomach. This inflammation not only affects the gastric mucous membrane but also extends to the muscle layer of the stomach. This is shown by the fact that both the white and black streaks extend from the pupillary margin fully to the iris-wreath.

The complaint here was: severe burning sensation in the stomach which can also include the abdomen, since the intestine also participates in the condition.

Note particularly the elongated black signs which begin at 38′ in the iris-wreath and extend with interruptions as far as the iris-rim. These signs are enclosed within two white zig-zag lines. The zig-zag form of these signs suggests the presence of inflammatory adhesions, whereas the black signs indicate tissue loss affecting the bile-ducts. (A)

Since this case is a typical example of cirrhosis and calcification, it should be stated that it is not so much the condition of stomach and intestine which would lead to ultimate dissolution as the hepatic cirrhosis, which is more important. Severe disturbance of the liver is shown by the flattening of the iris-rim from 35′ to 40′. The white ring in the sixth minor zone is the sign for calcification (cholesterosis ring).

The case record dating from 1938 states: The patient's father died from a stroke at the age of 59 years and his mother died from cancer of the liver at the age of 58 years. The patient himself, who was 72 years old in 1938, weighed 126 lbs. and was 1.74 metres in height. From the age of 18 years he had complained continually of stomach pains and vomiting. Haemorrhage had aiso occurred from time to time.

At the first consultation the symptoms were: sense of pressure in the stomach together with severe burning pains, retching and salivation. From 1938 to 1943 the patient felt well for long periods but with some interruptions. In 1939 he was still active in his earlier vocation as a locksmith.

The patient died in 1943. The death certificate recorded cancer of the liver. That the diagnosis of cancer of the liver is correct is not questioned, but that should not assume that the same signs must be present with every case of hepatic cancer as are to be seen in this iris.

Iris-26   **Female: 58 years—left iris**

Consideration of this iris shows almost the same state of the stomach zone as in Iris-1.

As a consequence of faulty nutrition, even worse signs are to be found in the second minor zone, as shown by the large dilatations of the iris-wreath and the black signs. The presence of white deposits in the fifth minor zone arises because of the deficient processing of nutritional materials, indicated by the signs in the first and second minor zones (as in Iris-1 and Iris-2), together with limitation of the motor powers suggested by the signs in the third and fourth minor zones. However, the signs in these zones are much worse than those in Iris-1, showing large and dark lacunae.

The general weakness affecting the muscle tissues has probably developed because the vegetative nervous system is less oversensitive and exhausted than is the case with Iris-1 (shown by the compact state of the iris-fibres). The large lacunae seen in Iris-26 suggest that the patient overstresses herself physically. Compare the difference in pupillary size shown by iris-pictures 1, 2 and 26. In Iris-1 the pupil is too large and indicates nervous exhaustion. In Iris-2 the pupil is too small, suggesting nerve over-stimulation. In Iris-26 a better equilibrium of the nervous system is shown by the large first and second minor zones, in which there is also an absence of inflammation signs.

The patient with Iris-2 has severe constipation, whereas the patient with Iris-26 tends to suffer diarrhoea. In this case a condition of fermentative dyspepsia affects the small intestine, from which much toxic material is absorbed, disturbing elimination through the kidneys and skin.

This patient is also predisposed to moist eruptions, which may cover the whole body if for any reason intestinal or renal excretion is disturbed, and more especially if materials having an allergic response are taken up into the blood stream. Exposure to strong sunshine can also provoke the eruption. I have frequently relieved such skin eruptions quite rapidly by treatment of the intestinal function and skin. Under longer treatment the white ring in the fifth minor zone can also disappear.

Iris-1:   Lymphatic constitution with nervous weakness but good function of intestines and skin.

Iris-2:   Lymphatic constitution with over-stimulation of the vegetative nerves and poor intestinal, renal and skin function.

Iris-26: Lymphatic constitution, good nervous system, pathological condition of the intestine, poor skin and kidney function.

As stated above, a patient with an iris like No. 26 tends to general overstress of the body vitality, but can in fact endure this overstress better than those whose irides are similar to Iris-1 or Iris-2. In this respect I give the substance of a conversation with an inspector of carrier-pigeons.

Carrier-pigeon inspectors, of which there are three or four in the whole of Germany, are required by the carrier-pigeon society to check and examine the young pigeons for their suitability. The inspectors are in a sense irisdiagnosticians, although their irisdiagnosis is limited to a differentiation of the pigeons eyes according to the looseness or compactness of the iris-texture. The young birds which show a loose and particularly coarse structure are regarded as suitable, whereas those which show a compact texture are considered unsuitable. The inspector to whom I spoke could not say what he saw in the pigeons' eyes. Only as he showed me several young pigeons from stock regarded as suitable or unsuitable, was it apparent that the single differential feature was the loose or compact texture of the iris.

This agrees with our interpretation. One can appreciate that pigeons showing a coarse texture of the iris will possess a similar coarse structure of the tissues and will be able for a time to endure excessive strain, whereas the birds showing a fine iris texture have no great capacity to call upon, since the finer body structure simply has no such reserve.

Nervous stress also contributes to this behaviour. Patients with a coarse iris-texture are not aware of the state of exhaustion until they reach the point of collapse, whereas those showing a fine textural iris experience an anxiety response before the stress situation develops and find that the nervous system will not endure so strong a stress.

The large dilatation of the iris-wreath at 60′ (A) indicates a condition of the large intestine involving the vegetative nervous system. It is to be considered in relation to the signs in the second and third major zones of the brain area, as well as to the signs placed diametrically opposite at 30′ in the ciliary zones.

The displaced sign at 29-30′ in the second major zone refers to the suprarenal gland (B). Such a large, suprarenal sign with a small black kidney sign raises the question of contracted kidney. The black sign at 30′ in the third major zone (C) suggests damage to the leg. There is here a disharmony between the head and the feet, producing giddiness and disturbed equilibrium (see the harmonic conjunction lines in *Fundamental Basis of Irisdiagnosis* of T. Kriege).

The large dilatation of the iris-wreath at 15′ (D) shows distension of the colon with consequent pressure upon the diaphragm. This in turn can produce cardiac symptoms.

On considering the large dark lacuna in the heart area at 10-14′ (E), it may be assumed that the disturbances of equilibrium are associated with anxiety conditions and are aggravated by emotional excitement.

The small black signs lying immediately below the white arc-line at 10′ (F) are signs of valvular defects consequent upon a suppurative condition of the tonsils or acute joint rheumatism. Likewise the small oblique black signs adjacent to the lower border of the heart sign at 15′ (G), taken together with the small black oval signs, indicate the presence of adhesions affecting the heart and pericardium.

The long black kidney sign at 33' (H) in the second major zone indicates tissue damage, and together with the large displaced suprarenal sign at 29-30' (B) is responsible for the disturbances in water-balance.

The signs in the brain areas, seen at 55-60' and 2-6' (J) diametrically opposite the renal and suprarenal areas, suggest involvement of the central nervous system in relation to the pituitary, mid-brain and vegetative nervous functions.

White radial signs at 24-26' and 33-38' (K), which extend as far as the iris-margin in the areas for anus, vagina and lower abdomen, suggest the presence of a chronic eruption in the form of a weeping eczema. The dark signs at 37' and 39' in the third major zone indicate chronic vaginal and rectal catarrh of long standing.

The case record states as follows:

Housewife, 58 years of age, the fourth child of seven, married with six children.

Father died at 83 years of age from pneumonia. Mother died at 78 years of age from senile decline.

Earlier illness: At 14 years of age always developed nettlerash on exposure to the evening mist. Suffered many attacks of tonsillitis during childhood. Menstruation did not commence until 18 years of age. At the age of 40 years developed joint rheumatism which lasted four weeks, then spasms of the gall-bladder appeared. At 46 years of age was bedridden for a long time with pneumonia (note the signs at 15-20' in the third major zone). Suffered periodic bouts of intense rheumatic pains throughout 30 years.

The symptoms recorded at the first consultation (9.9.38) were: a moist eruption on the face and over the whole body for four weeks following the healing of an open leg condition. Several physicians diagnosed sunburn, eczema, eruption. The eruption was healed within four weeks. Further treatment was given until February 1939 and there was no return up to that time. In July, 1947 the patient again came under care for an irritating eczema of the lower abdomen. Up to that time there had been no return of the eruption.

Compared with Iris-26, the gastro-intestinal zone appears too white (inflammation and passive congestion), with strong contractions and dilatations as well as black signs to be seen. In the blood and muscle zones however, the lacunae are less conspicuously large, but there are more black signs denoting organ damage and very dark closed lacunae.

In particular, there are signs of damage to such organs as kidney, suprarenal gland, pancreas, heart and aorta. This is not merely weakness of function but definite organ damage, so that every functional disturbance which appears must be considered serious. Vegetative dysfunction arises in consequence of the suprarenal condition (signs at 29' in the third minor zone—A) and include symptoms of a cramp-like nature: intestinal colic, circulatory conditions affecting the heart and involving conduction and myocardial function (heart signs at 9-15' and aortic signs at 6' in the third minor zone).

The condition of the pancreas (dark signs at 20-23' in the third and fourth minor zones—B) shows a possibility of glycosuria and even if this is not yet evident, there will be digestive disturbances giving rise to intestinal symptoms, from flatulence to colic.

The tendency to catarrh of mucous and serous membranes is shown by the small white flakes in the sixth minor zone, which considered with the black signs in this zone, raises the question of a tubercular disposition. In this connection, note particularly the areas for lungs and pleurae (12-18', 43-50'—sixth minor zone) as well as the kidney sign at 32' in the third and fourth minor zones (C).

Iris-27 thus shows more organ damage, whereas the predominant feature of Iris-26 is the muscle weakness. That of Iris-2 is the general cramping, and of Iris-1 the nervous weakness.

Apart from the many pointed and rounded contractions and dilatations, the first major zone shows strong contraction of the iris-wreath generally, which at 5' and 10' almost reaches the pupillary margin. The black signs within the wreath-zone at this location, together with those seen diametrically opposite at 35-40', are defect-signs indicating extensive ulceration of the posterior wall of the stomach. These ulcerative changes have produced a constriction of the organ (hour-glass stomach).

However, the condition is not limited to the stomach, but has extended to involve the transverse colon at a point immediately before the splenic flexure, as shown by the two constrictions of the wreath at 5′ and 7′ (D). These indications of adhesions affecting the large intestine have been confirmed by radiography. The straight course of the iris-wreath between 60′ and 15′ (allowing for the interposition of the two constrictions) indicates ptosis of the transverse colon and also suggests the possibility of a dropped stomach. This however, cannot be confirmed in view of the small gastro-intestinal area.

Observing both sides of the iris-wreath at 5′, it is seen that on each side the sign runs to a point enclosing a dark spot, suggesting that the condition has healed (D). At 9′ the process has not yet resolved, since the dark sign extends to the iris-rim and widens as it does so (E). This suggests that the symptoms from the stomach refer up to the neck.

The closed lacuna at 6′ in the fourth minor zone, between the two constriction signs just described is to be regarded as an aortic sign (F). Also note the left ear-bladder line.

Consider now the large dark, but not closed, lacuna at 2-5′, which also widens as it extends outwards to the iris-rim (G). From this, it might be assumed that the circulation to the head is poor and more especially that there is an encumbrance of the mid-brain. This sign lies diametrically opposite to the kidney sign at 32′, suggesting that the cerebral condition is also influenced by the renal disturbance.

In relation to this, consider the signs referring to the endocrine system, in particular: the closed lacuna at 59′ in the second major zone (hypophysis), the tissue-weakness sign at 29′ in the second major zone (suprarenal), the closed lacuna with tissue damage at 22′ (pancreas), the long dark sign in the second and third major zone at 25′ (gonads), together with the associated signs at 37′ on the ear-bladder line (H). From these indications it is clear that dysfunction of these organs results in a severe stress affecting the nervous system as well as the blood circulation (see heart signs at 10-15′ in the second major zone). The lymphatic system is also implicated, as is shown by the white signs extending outwards from the iris-wreath to the periphery, especially between 25′ and 50′.

The multiform signs seen between 38′ and 45′, extending over the second and third major zones refer to the vertebral column and indicate encumbrance affecting the back. This involvement of the spinal nerves is to be considered together with the signs for the genital organs and bladder already discussed.

The stress affecting the endocrine and circulatory systems does not appear as specific symptoms, but underlies the general state of health and must be taken into account in assessing the acute conditions presented. The symptoms complained of concern the stomach and intestines, with special emphasis on the rectum. The small black signs at 33-37' in the third major zone, which appear to press apart the white radial lines into an arc-shape (tumour sign), indicate a severe degree of venous stasis affecting the rectum (haemorrhoids with tissue degeneration). The white wisp signs reaching to the iris-rim suggest exudation through the skin. The existence of such signs is a positive indication to undertake a rectal inspection, since there may be a concealed malignant ulcer (J).

Case record notes: The patient is a country postman, 47 years of age, married with no children. The first consultation raised the following problems: liver and gall-bladder symptoms, adhesions of stomach and intestines, gastroptosis, haemorrhoids and anal irritation.

Iris-28   **Male: 40 years—left iris**

Comparing this iris with Iris-2, it is seen that the first major zone in both is very small. The pupil is likewise too small (over-stimulation of the vegetative nervous system). However, this zone is not so white as in Iris-2. The almost black colouring shows the absence of inflammation and because of the poor circulation, induration and atrophy affecting the tissues, there is a reduced functional capacity with insufficient nutrition and absorption of toxic material from the intestine.

The white ring surrounding the first major zone, representing the iris-wreath, shows lymphatic stasis, which is further affected by the weakness of the heart and circulation (note heart signs at 10-17'—A). The functional activity of the skin and kidneys is good, so that no particular disturbance arises from these organs.

The cause of the presenting conditions lies in the dysfunction of the nervous system and the alimentary absorption of toxic materials. The latter produces auto-intoxication affecting all

91

tissues, shown by the overall dark to black point-like signs. Such signs arise from unresolved disturbances, as with Iris-2.

When lymph nodes (lymph glands) become inflamed and swollen from the absorbed toxic material and the condition remains unresolved, they gradually harden. Thus, following inflammation (increased activity) there is induration (reduced activity), in which the function of the lymphocytes to break down toxic material is no longer performed. Ultimately, no more lymphocytes are produced and there is a progressive reduction in the number circulating. The organism finally deteriorates from auto-intoxication.

Referring to the long dark sign with the adjoining white sign at 35′ in the second and third major zones (B), the chronic catarrh of the rectum indicated arises on a background of chronic gastro-intestinal catarrh and circulatory stasis. The cardio-vascular weakness already presupposes a condition of venous stasis affecting the lower part of the body, leading to restricted blood vessels and haemorrhoids. The added condition of constipation results in extended disturbances, especially where the general way of life is sedentary.

Civilised man takes his nourishment in a form which does not provide sufficient bulk material for the lumen of the intestine (fat, white bread, sugar, fruit and vegetable juices). Consequently, the intestine must overcontract in order to propel the small content. This condition already affects the small intestine, but when in the large intestine with its still greater lumen the fluid content is absorbed, then almost nothing remains to facilitate the normal function of the colon. If, in addition, the intake of fluid is too small, then at the end of the alimentary process the final residue consists of 'coffee-bean' or pea-shaped particles.

Note especially the thick white iris-wreath between 10′ and 20′, suggesting a condition of coronary sclerosis (A).

The following notes appear on the case record: The patient is an official, 40 years old, married, no children. Earlier illness: an attack of measles during childhood. Some years ago suffered from suppuration of the tonsils. Military doctors established the existence of adhesions in the abdominal cavity.

The following symptoms and conditions were recorded at the first consultation: pain and swelling in the region of the liver, focal infection from granuloma, constipation and haemorrhoids.

On the whole, the texture of this iris is to be regarded as compact. From the small pupil and the size of the first major zone, which is too small, a disturbed condition of the central and vegetative nervous systems is indicated. The person with such a condition never achieves repose. Since the signs appear so prominently in the right iris, hereditary influences are implied.

The thick white surrounding border of the iris-wreath shows that considerable stress affects the lymphatic system from inflammation of the intestines. The white lines radiating outwards from the wreath extend to the peripheral iris-rim. The most prominent lines are to be found in organ areas: forehead (7-8'), throat (11-18'), abdomen (24-28'), ovary and abdominal cavity (33-37') and thorax (40-50'), which suggests that the conditions are most significant (A).

The conditions are evidenced by neuralgic pains, especially as burning pains and dry catarrh affecting the throat, nose, mouth, vagina and bladder. The anus is not free from these symptoms since the area for anus and rectum in the left iris shows similar prominent signs.

The patient is a small, thin person, whose face is distorted by pain. She has never felt well and suffers the symptoms described above. For years she has been under treatment for burning pains in the vagina, with and without cautery, but all without success. The best response was always obtained by homoeopathy, but even with this treatment complete freedom from pain has not yet been achieved, since the nervous dysfunction is too considerable and arises from hereditary factors.

Dark to black points are seen especially in the sixth minor zone, suggesting induration of the lymphatics and a tendency to focal infection. But in this case, there is not such a picture of total intoxication as is seen in Iris-28. Instead, there is more the picture of neuralgia.

With Iris-28, there would be danger from all surgical operations, which would never be without complications and usually subsequent demise. In the case of Iris-29, however, foci of infection need to be removed, although such measures seldom bring any improvement in the symptoms.

Iris-32 is that of the patient's son. In spite of the compact iris of the mother and an almost healthy iris of the father, that of the son is very bad.

Comparing Iris-29 with the preceding Iris-28, the latter may be likened to a swamp in which moss proliferates between the puddles of water, whereas the former appears like a dried landscape in which vegetation is no longer present. In reality it is just so. Iris-28 represents a person of bloated appearance, torpid, lacking adequate sensitivity to painful stimuli and without reactivity, whereas Iris-29 represents one who is thin, dried up, irritable, excitable and senses everything too acutely. Iris-28 shows a lymphatic system which is completely static and full of debris, whereas in Iris-29 it is dried out and empty.

The case sheet records the following details: Housewife, 46 years of age, the third child of three siblings, of which one died from peritonitis at the age of 55 years and one sister is still living. The patient is married with one child. The father died from senile weakness at 96 years of age. The mother died at 60 years of age from cancer of the throat.

The history recorded earlier diseases of whooping cough and nervous dyspepsia. At the first consultation there was: inflammation of the stomach mucous membrane with excessive secretion of stomach acid, nervous disturbance affecting one organ after another and irritation of the left kidney, dry catarrh of the nose and throat, dry cough, burning sensation in the vagina after micturition and in the anus.

The preceding irides—26, 27, 28 and 29—all show evidence of an allergic disposition. The attacks of nettlerash suffered by patient-26 are without question of an allergic nature. Likewise, the stomach ulcers suffered by patient-27 may be based on allergic responses. Equally with patients 28 and 29, the conditions appearing have basically the same cause. It is all a question of the interaction of differing constitutions with their varied dispositions and the different ways in which the presenting conditions have developed. Just as different kinds of materials may produce the same allergic response, so a variety of presenting symptoms may result and require a variety of homoeopathic medicines for the cure.

The border of the first minor zone is too sharply defined and also too light in colour. These signs indicate that stomach pains, heartburn and salivation are present together.

The second minor zone is too narrow and contains many black signs, indicating the probability of frequent attacks of intestinal inflammation during childhood, and that now the diet contains too little roughage and so leads to constipation. Also in such cases there is generally too little drunk. The dilatation of the iris-wreath at 10-15' shows the existence of Roemhelds syndrome.

The heart area, at 10-15' of the second major zone in the left iris, may in certain cardiac conditions extend far beyond these limits. In this case, every sign is to be regarded as indicating a disturbance of the heart. If signs relative to other organs intrude into this area, then there is a pathological condition of the other organ, e.g. stomach, intestine, lungs, etc. Cardiac disturbances are generally the secondary consequence of other conditions and in turn, disturbances of other organs may arise as a result of the cardiac dysfunction.

I have chosen iris illustration No. 30 for the reason that on superficial examination no signs are to be seen in the heart area. However, observation of the dark fifth and sixth minor zones shows the presence of small points, especially between 40' and 50' (A), and these indications immediately raise the question of a focal infection. Since the consequences of this condition are infection of the blood with inflammation of the endocardium and cardiac defects, then one cannot help but examine the heart area more closely. It will be found that in the second major zone between 10' and 15', small dark islands are seen between the white lines (B). These are signs showing that the heart has been involved through the infection. If the main symptoms for stomach and intestinal disturbances also exist (the most severe pains probably affect the back) then cardiac complaints will have appeared already.

The iris here portrayed shows a sensitive type (Empfindungstyp), subject to nerve pains which can affect the whole body. As already stated, in irides such as these, the slightest variation in the normal course of the iris tissue-structure should be noted, as for example, the downward deviation of the contraction rings at 30' in the leg area, indicating a condition of stasis (C). The separation of the iris fibres at 35-37' in the fourth minor zone together with the small black signs at the same location which extend outwards as far as the iris-rim, suggest dilatation of the ampulla and a condition of haemorrhoids (D).

The increased whiteness at 37' and 38' in the second and third major zones indicates catarrh of the bladder, and the small white oblique line in the fifth minor zone a stricture of the urethra (E). The contraction rings in this segment are also interrupted, suggesting cramplike disturbances.

The thick white lines at 42' and 43' which extend from the pupil to the iris-margin indicate an acute condition of the nerves in the back (F). The small black points, which have been described above, signify the existence of granuloma or suppurating foci, which as partly active will disseminate, and partly closed off give rise to no special appearances.

The case record notes the following:
Housewife, 32 years of age, the fourth child of nine siblings, married with one child.
Previous illnesses: measles and nasal diphtheria during childhood. An operation on the appendix two years previously and an operation for uterine tumour and prolapse ten weeks previously.
Symptoms recorded at the first consultation:
Pains in the back which had been present for some time.
Headaches, especially in the temple.
Epigastric pressure accompanied by salivation.
A sensation of throat obstruction for which the patient had already twice undertaken a cure for tapeworm.
Cardiac anxiety, bleeding gums, suppurative foci at the roots of the teeth. Pains in the rectum, constipation.
Diagnosis: Suppurative frontal and maxillary sinusitis.
　　　　Bleeding and inflammation of the gums.
　　　　Pharyngeal catarrh with suppuration.
　　　　Haemorrhoids.

Iris-31　　　　　　　　　　　　　**Female: 32 years—left iris**

Observe the large pupil, the small first major zone and the sharply defined line of the iris-wreath. The area for rectum at 36-37' in the third major zone strikes the attention immediately.

Everything points to chronic catarrh of the stomach and intestines. In addition, the signs at 20' and 40' in the third and fourth minor zones suggest pancreatic insufficiency with a diabetic tendency (A).

Adjacent to the iris-wreath at 29' a small black sign is seen in the suprarenal area (B). This is a sign denoting severe injury to the suprarenal gland, involving disturbance of the vegetative nervous system. The conditions of these organs affect each other, in which case the various symptoms appearing now here, now there, will not be cured if these connections are not appreciated.

The heart sign at 12-16' should be regarded as an open lacuna, since the white bordering lines are not closed. The suggested myocardial weakness has probably arisen as the result of the conditions described above (C).

Immediately below the heart weakness sign (lacuna) two white zig-zag lines are to be seen coursing outwards (D). These indicate that the symptom of cardiac palpitation arises especially after exertion. The patient is unable to sustain effort because of heart weakness. In addition, several small black point-like signs appear within the lacuna. Similar signs are to be seen elsewhere in the iris, especially in the fifth and sixth minor zones. They indicate focal infection and make the patient's condition unbearable. As is well known, focal infections give rise to rheumatic pains. These symptoms may be deduced from the presence of white clouds in the fourth and fifth minor zones, especially adjacent to the heart sign at 12-15' (C). Consequently, the cardiac symptoms are also influenced by the weather. If such connections are not appreciated by the practitioner, his treatment will never be successful. Every medicine chosen to meet the foregoing conditions will merely relieve individual symptoms for a short time, but not achieve a cure (note skin and kidneys).

Several signs in the third major zone are quite striking, apart from the white clouds at 12' and 15', especially at 23', 25' and 29'. This is the area for peritoneum and ovary. In this area, the iris-margin has a grey colouring. In addition, a long dark sign beginning as a small black dot at the iris-wreath (28') extends outwards to the iris-margin. This dark sign is to be regarded as an ovary-sign and indicates an old chronic condition. The adjacent white clouds are the expression of a persisting inflammation (E).

At 37' a white zig-zag line is seen which extends from the iris-wreath to the iris-margin and suggests a condition of nerve inflammation with pains affecting the bladder and urethra. The quite short white oblique line within the zig-zag line also indicates injury (F).

How are these signs to be interpreted? Consider the grey margin of the iris between 55' and 7' which also has a definite silvery sheen. This sign always suggests the presence of scalp irritation and loss of hair, generally caused by certain excesses in youth. This accords with the grey iris-rim at 23-29' and with the ovary sign. Together with the bladder sign, we have the cause for many complaints. The considerable weakness shown by the large pupil may now also be understood.

Let us remain with these signs for the time being. Note that the iris-wreath in the lower half of the iris lies nearer to the pupil than in the upper half. This accordingly implies that the stomach and intestines are displaced upwards by some condition in the lower abdominal cavity. It may be assumed that the cause is an ovarian tumour, even though pressure on both sides of the iris-wreath at 15-20' and 37-45' also indicates a swelling of the pancreas. A sign for enlargement of the pancreas may indeed be recognised at 20' and 40' in the second major zone adjacent to the iris-wreath (A).

The two small apparently black signs at 28' in the third major zone and at 29' at the iris-wreath are in fact brown toxin-flecks, which as such are without significance. When, however, they lie at or near organ-signs, then it may be taken that the conditions are always difficult to resolve.

The white clouds at 45' and 48' in the third major zone in the sector for the face suggest a latent condition of naso-pharyngeal catarrh (G).

Now consider the two white signs at 12' and 15' in the third major zone (C). Although these indicate an influence affecting the heart, they also suggest a catarrhal state of the lungs. In relation to this, the small black points in the sixth minor zone at 15-20' suggest local intoxications from foci in the rib area. As with dental granuloma, these may give rise to secondary symptoms.

To judge from the left iris alone and without taking into account the signs in the right iris, the development of the total condition would be as follows: Serious encumbrance from stomach and intestinal disturbances. From sexual excesses, aggravation of the general condition by inflammatory reactions with tissue destruction and focal infections, leading to severe cardiac stress and involvement of the nervous and endocrine systems, in turn producing mento-emotional stress.

The case-card records as follows—

Domestic servant, 32 years of age, single.

Earlier illnesses: inflammation of the knee joint at the age of 17 years, inflammation of the hip joint at the age of 24 years. Two years later, suppuration of the glands of the neck on the left side.

Symptoms and conditions at the first consultation—

Suppuration of the ear involving four weeks of specialist treatment. During the past 14 days, severe stomach pains on waking every morning which reduce by midday. Moderate palpitations of the heart on exertion.

Iris-32   **Child: 10 years—left iris**

This iris illustrates the lymphatic constitution, the exudative diathesis. The pupil is too large, suggesting nerve weakness. The first and second minor zones are wider in the ventral sector with several large dilatations. White signs denoting inflammatory conditions are numerous.

The iris-wreath is clearly identified as a white indented ring. From 10′ to 45′ the white clouds in the third major zone extend outwards to the iris-margin and show the presence of a moist eruption. The links between the skin elimination and the chronic gastro-intestinal catarrh are clearly seen. It is not merely the eruptions which are symptomatic of an exudative diathesis, but also the glandular swelling and the catarrh of the mucous membranes which are frequently presented by this patient.

The large closed weakness-sign (lacuna) in the heart area at 13′ to 16′ in this picture is related to the severe exhaustion of the patient (A). Indeed, the whole of the second major zone is covered with lacunae, thus suggesting a bloated spongy body in which the entire musculature is exhausted.

The composition of the blood is very poor. The large heart sign could easily lead to the conclusion that considerable cardiac enlargement must be present, but this is not the case. The heart may well be somewhat dilated from exhaustion, but it can never be assumed that the size of the heart itself is to be inferred from the size of the heart-sign. This large sign indicates only that the power of the heart is weakened.

There is a potential danger of heart failure in any acute febrile condition, such as pneumonia. It will be necessary for any practitioner to prescribe not only the medicines necessary to relieve the acute condition, but also from the outset to include agents for the heart and circulation.

Note the small closed lacunae at 19, 21, 25, 29 and 33 in the second major zone (B). These are signs in the third minor zone and indicate resolved or compensated conditions. The sign at 21', which looks like a square suspended from the lacuna, refers to the pancreas, which at this position suggests a tendency to diabetes. Similarly, the large kidney and suprarenal signs indicate a tubercular tendency (C).

Referring to the iris picture of the patient's mother (No. 29), it can be seen that a basically bad heredity has become even worse. Only by long-term treatment with constitutional medicines would it be possible to achieve something in this case, to prevent the potential disease condition.

Considering the heart sign more closely, it is seen that there is a large upper and a smaller lower section (A). The upper part is to be regarded as a direct heart sign, whereas the lower section refers to the pericardium. In this patient, there is a tendency to pericardial effusion. Within the larger sector there are some small black points, indicating that the heart valves have become incompetent and are no longer equal to any increased stress.

Note particularly the almost black sign at 57' and 58' in the second major zone (D). It indicates a serious state of the pituitary gland, which as the leading endocrine gland influences the entire internal secretory system with its hormones. The sign in the second major zone at 3', the pineal gland (E), and also at 18', the thymus gland (F), explain why this patient developed gigantism. At 16 years of age the boy was 1.88 m. in height. From that point the long-growth remained unchanged. On call-up for military service, heart weakness was established.

The following appears on the case card:
The patient is a 10 year old schoolboy (Iris illustration No. 29 shows the mother's iris.)
The father is a large and powerfully built man and has had no diseases worth mentioning. Of the father's relatives, one sister died

during childbirth. Of the mother's relatives, one sister is still living, the other sister died at the age of 55 years from peritonitis after an intestinal perforation following colonic irrigation.

Grandparents: the paternal grandfather died at the age of 76 years, the paternal grandmother is 84 years old and still alive. The maternal grandfather died of old age at 96 years, and the maternal grandmother died at the age of 60 years from cancer of the throat.

Earlier illnesses: contracted all the usual childhood infections. Between 1937 and 1945 the patient was treated at variable intervals for different conditions. Symptoms arising from chill appeared repeatedly, including bronchial catarrh, inflammation of the tonsils with swollen glands, nasal and pharyngeal catarrh. Diarrhoea was especially prominent, the patient suffering from it almost continually.

Iris-33   **Male: 38 years—left iris**

Note the first major zone. It is too small and too dark. This patient would be diagnosed in a hospital clinic as having pyloric tumours and referred for operative treatment. This condition is to be seen from the right iris.

The whole organism has been affected by this chronic condition of stomach and intestine of many years standing, as may be seen from the intensely white appearance of the second major zone in the nasal quadrants (30-60'). This shows the existence of inflammatory conditions arising on a rheumatic basis.

From the prominent white zig-zag lines at 20' (spleen line = pain line), it may be taken that the patient suffers intense pain. The dark sign at 20-25' in the third major zone, enclosed by white arc-lines extending outwards from the second major zone, indicates swelling of the spleen (A). Intense pain affecting the back may also be deduced from the interrupted white nerve rings between 36' and 42', as well as from the intensely white radial lines in the same area (B).

Similar interruption of the nerve rings can be seen in the heart area at 10-15', suggesting that cramp-like disturbances affect the heart. A large and almost dark heart sign is seen at 12-15' (C). It does not have the appearance of a typical lacuna with two white enclosing arc-lines, but is bordered below by a thick white straight line which gives the heart sign something of a wedge shape. The upper bordering white line is quite short and above the sign the fibres in the second major zone as far as 10 ' are loosely structured. These signs are found in conditions where circulatory disturbance of the myocardium exists (coronary sclerosis) (C).

The signs described up to this point indicate conditions which affect each other: severe gastro-intestinal disturbance, portal congestion (liver-spleen stasis) and total circulatory stress especially affecting the heart. From this arises narrowing of the coronary vessels and nutritional insufficiency affecting the myocardium (heart muscle weakness), stasis in the legs shown by the white clouds in the foot area, and haemorrhoids (small dark points at 35 ' in the third major zone) (D).

The dark open lacuna seen in the second major zone at 29 ' is a suprarenal sign. From its influence upon the vegetative nervous system, disturbances of this gland affect the blood circulation (E).

The long dark sign at 3 ' extending outwards from the second into the third major zone, together with the outward deviation of the white nerve ring at the same location, indicate the presence of stasis and swelling in the area of the mid-brain (F). This disturbance is connected with the kidney sign at 32 ' in the second and third major zones. The small black sign in this area indicates tissue damage (nephrosclerosis). The large, white surrounding oval extending from the iris-wreath to the third major zone suggests a persisting inflammatory condition (G).

The bladder sign at 37 ' should be interpreted in relation to the oblique white line at 25 '. The latter indicates injury to the left testicle with tissue damage, as shown by the small black sign. Consider the ureter (H).

In the area for the back between 38 ' and 44 ' in the second and third major zones the nerve rings are interrupted a number of times, and between the winding white radial fibres a quite straight line is seen which goes from 41 ' at the iris-margin to the small black streak inside the iris-wreath (J). This indicates a severe condition of the spinal column. Small dark signs are also present. These or similar signs in the back area are typical of multiple sclerosis and although no symptoms may yet be apparent, it shows a potential danger. At 50 ' and 51 ' the nerve rings are broken through by a longish black sign, suggesting a disturbance of the nasal sinuses (K). The extension of the white radial lines as far as the iris-margin indicates the presence of a chronic nasal catarrhal discharge.

On the case record is noted:
Mechanic, single, 38 years old.
Pyloric tumours diagnosed in hospital.
Symptoms reported at the first consultation: stomach pains, vomiting of food two hours after the meal. Heart symptoms with spasms. Pain and irritation of the anus.
Diagnosis: pyloric obstruction, haemorrhoids, cardiac dilatation, calcification of the coronary vessels.
Surgical treatment advised.

Iris-34   **Female: 17 years—left iris**

The first major zone is too small and contains several signs of disturbance. A striking feature is that this zone appears to be almost square-shaped and is narrower below than above. This raises the question of a possible tumour formation in the lower abdomen.

In this typically compact iris-structure the white clouds in the second and third major zones are especially prominent. This shows muscle and joint rheumatism. The heart area, which in this case extends from 8′ to 16′ and out over the third major zone, is also surrounded by white clouds. This large and somewhat loose-textured sign (A) with the white clouds indicates a rheumatic inflammation of the myocardium and the surrounding tissues. Within this large sign a small closed lacuna is to be found at 14′ in the third minor zone. Within the upper angle of the lacuna is a small black sign. The fact that the lacuna is closed suggests that the valvular lesion is compensated. It is not so with the adjacent sign in the fourth minor zone which is still not enclosed by white arc-lines and accordingly indicates an inflammatory and atrophic process affecting this heart valve. The small black sign shows the presence of tissue destruction, while the increased intensity of the whiteness immediately above is the indication for a persisting acute inflammation.

The closed heart sign at 14′ in the third minor zone probably developed from the diphtheria at 11 years of age. Note the sign for previous diphtheria at 45-50′ in the mouth and throat area. The iris colouring generally is too white in the ciliary zones, but lacking the prominently white iris-wreath seen in iris-35. This accordingly suggests that the present condition of joint rheumatism does not arise from a gastro-intestinal disturbance but from focal infection, which on the basis of a labile nervous system produces the symptoms and conditions. How are these connections derived?

The case history records inflammation of the heart valves following diphtheria at 11 years of age. The severe damage to heart and circulation probably resulted in insufficient nutrition of the tissues and the commencement of destructive processes.

Consider the thick white wavy line at 47′ which extends outwards over the second and third major zones showing two arcs directed below. This sign-complex indicates swelling of the neck. Similarly, the white radial lines at 49′ and 50′ have arcs directed above, showing that the disturbance extends as far as the maxilla. Within this area small black signs are seen in the third major zone. These indicate suppurative foci and the dilatation in the third major zone suggests swelling of the tonsils. The white line at 47′ in the third major zone is to be regarded as a laryngeal sign. The large white cloud in this same area indicates the presence of an acute state. (B)

When similar black signs are seen at 15-20′ in the third major zone other foci are also indicated, especially since white arc-lines are also to be found, suggesting an old pleurisy which produced adhesions and dessication of the exudate (C).

Although the signs may be apparent and the patient afterwards questioned accordingly, it does not follow that a condition will be confirmed. Probably the existence of a chronic cough will be admitted and radiography may show ulcerations in the pleural areas. Generally speaking, the patient does not remember that she had a condition affecting the pleura.

The long dark sign at 26′ in the second major zone with the adjacent white cloud at 27′ suggests a state of suprarenal irritation. Likewise with the sign at 31′ and 33′ in the second major zone (kidney sign) (D). These two signs, kidney and suprarenal, develop as dark signs in contrast to the remainder of the iris after resolution of an acute inflammatory condition. If healing takes place after long duration of a condition involving severe damage to the organ, then a closed lacuna will be found. The upward displacement of the iris wreath in this area (31-33′) can arise from the disturbance affecting the last two organ conditions described if tumours develop.

On the case record is noted:

Housemaid, 17 years of age. Parents healthy.

Of the mother's relatives, one brother died from pneumonia, and another brother from sarcoma. The paternal grandfather died from pneumonia at the age of 65 years. The paternal grandmother suffered with a stomach ailment. The maternal grandfather suffered from asthma.

Earlier illnesses: Had measles during childhood. At the age of 11 years developed endocarditis following diphtheria. One year ago again developed endocarditis from focal infection as well as rheumatic pains in the joints.

Current complaint: Acute joint rheumatism over the previous three weeks.

Iris-35   **Female: 60 years—left iris**

In this iris, the peaked expansions of the gastro-intestinal zone between 7′ and 27′ with their enclosed black signs are readily apparent (descending colon). These signs indicate the presence of chronic intestinal catarrh extending as far as the anus at 35′ where a long black sign is seen commencing at the iris-wreath and widening towards the iris-margin (haemorrhoids). The bunched white lines at the periphery show irritation and burning of the anus. The prominent white zig-zag radial at this location is a sign for violent pain and inflammation (A).

The white colouring of the iris-wreath in the sector for small intestine, 37′ to 55′, and for transverse colon, 55′ to 7′, shows inflammatory conditions affecting the intestinal tract with irritation of the lymphatic system (dysbacteria with auto-intoxication).

Now consider the dark to black sign at 11-15′ in the second major zone, consisting of two large dark signs with two small signs above. The two small signs may be regarded as closed lacunae, whereas the two larger signs should not be so considered. They each begin narrowly at the iris-wreath and have a wider base directed towards the iris-margin. Viewed together, these four signs indicate cardiac enlargement which has arisen from stressing a heart suffering from coronary sclerosis (B).

The picture of sclerosis of the coronary vessels is always to be observed in a subdivided heart sign. It is typically shown by a prominent dirty white, not sharp line bordering the heart sign at the iris wreath, as may be seen in this illustration (B).

The sign observed at 8-11′ in the third and fourth minor zones suggests that the aorta is also involved (C). However, since a high blood pressure is to be assumed where there is sclerosis, then the possibility of renal disease as the cause should be checked. Accordingly, special attention is given to the kidney areas in both irides, and if small black signs or honeycomb signs are found, then the possibility of contracted kidney should be considered.

Any suprarenal signs should also be noted, as seen here at 28′ and 29′ (D). At 29′ in the third minor zone a long and narrow black sign indicates a disturbance of the suprarenal body, involving destruction of the glandular tissue. Such a sign shows involvement of the vegetative nervous system (vegetative dystony), leading to over-contraction in the supporting organ-systems.

This disturbance has probably produced the sclerosis of the coronary vessels and the blood vessels generally, as well as the condition of angina pectoris. (Compare with iris illustration No. 34—focal infection). Because of this long-standing suprarenal disturbance, cure or improvement of the patient's condition is obstructed.

The development of the syndrome is probably as follows: intestinal infection leading to exhaustion of the body reserves, further aggravated by excessive stress and consequent collapse of the resistance organisation (lymph system). This in turn results in obstructive deposits within the vascular system and simultaneous collapse of the hormone system, which stands in direct relation to the vegetative nervous system. This involves the central nervous system.

Failure of the hormone system is to be seen not only from the signs of suprarenal disturbance, but also from the sign placed diametrically opposite at 57-58′ in the third major zone—the area for the pituitary gland (E). Also note the light arc-line at the iris-wreath between 22′ and 25′ (swelling of the pancreas), with the lighter colouring towards the iris-rim. The light cloud at 20′ in the second major zone shows inflammatory irritation of the pancreas and of the tissues surrounding the organ (F).

Observing the intensely white sign at 37-40′ (iris-wreath) and the dark signs in the same area, one can assume that the condition of the pancreas is related to some pathology involving the posterior wall of the stomach (G). This picture shows the obvious insidious cachexia.

That the patient should still be capable of work may be attributed to the existing healthy skin function (iris-rim). The grey peripheral margin between 50' and 10' suggests heavy deposits in the head and usually results in falling hair and scalp irritation.

On the case record is noted:

Housewife, 60 years of age, the second child of eight siblings, married with six children (one child died at 3 months of age from pneumonia, one child lived for only half a day).

The father died at the age of 43 years from asthma. The mother died at 74 years of age from cancer of the trachea.

Earlier illnesses: Measles. Cranial operation at the age of 20 years to relieve dreadful pains in the head. Uterine operation at 47 years of age and an operation of the eyelid-glands at 50 years.

At the first consultation the symptoms were: stomach and intestinal symptoms with strong flatulence, heart cramps, arteriosclerosis especially of the coronary vessels, anxiety state, buzzing in the ears. The patient had been treated in hospital for angina-pectoris.

Iris-36   **Female: 49 years—left iris**

This iris is that of a 49 year old housewife who came from hospital complaining of severe pain in the upper part of the right arm. At this location there was a suppurating ulcer of the bone marrow which had been opened and in spite of fourteen days treatment, the unbearable pain had not abated.

Iris examination immediately drew attention to the large dark signs at 20-24' in the second major zone of the left iris, relating to the tail of the pancreas (A). The assumption of disturbed sugar metabolism was confirmed by examination of the urine. Neither from the attending physician, nor in hospital, had there been any examination for sugar level. As the result of dietetic regulation, medicine and insulin, the urine became sugar-free, the severe pain rapidly receded and the wound closed quickly.

To return to the iris signs. Considering the large dark lacunae which cover almost half of the entire iris area, it is seen that all are open to the periphery. Since they extend as far as the fifth minor zone, considerable weakness in the state of the blood, muscle and bone generally is indicated. The large, dark sign at 20-24' in the second major zone (A) indicates functional insufficiency of the pancreas. The cause of many diseases, including that of the pancreas, originates in the digestive tract. The signs of disease in the first major zone confirm this.

In relation to this, note particularly the dark sign at 50' in the second major zone and the hardly visible closed lacuna within the white cloud at 19' (B). If the mouth-hand line (nutrition line) is emphasised so in the left iris, it may be assumed that there is faulty nutrition. Such patients are very taciturn and whatever is said is of significance. This patient answered only to questions and the husband had to provide the details.

The three large dark lacunae in the second major zone at 12-18' are to be regarded as heart signs (C). The condition indicated is one of general myocardial weakness and coronary sclerosis. The dark sign at 9' refers to the aorta (D). Since the iris-wreath in this sector adopts a markedly zig-zag course and deviates outwards, there will be symptoms of heartburn and flatulence (gastro-cardial syndrome).

Considerable weakness of the back is shown by the lacunae at 40-45' in the second major zone of the dorsal area (E). Taken with the signs at 8', remember the association of shoulder and lower back (shoulder-loin line = endurance line). Patients showing signs which emphasise this association are unable to perform much physical work—they can neither carry much, nor endure much. Patient-36 is small, stout and bloated in appearance.

The dark signs in the back area and the large heart signs lying diametrically opposite suggest that no great vital power is available. The treatment of such a patient must be very careful.

The dark sign at 47' in the area for throat and larynx is unfavourable in relation to the lungs (F). The white flakes seen in the third major zone at 8-17' and 40-50' indicate serous membrane catarrh affecting the thoracic organs. Together with the dark scurf-rim in the same segments, these signs indicate previously suppressed conditions.

Referring to the large dark sign at 28-31' in the second major zone (suprarenal—G), it can be seen that vegetative disturbances are a contributory factor in the general picture. Although the sign is large, it is only dark—not black, and thus shows that there is functional insufficiency without tissue destruction. The tendency towards honey-comb formation within the sign indicates functional incompetence from over-contraction or atrophic changes.

Special attention should be given to the white transversal in the leg area at 30-34′ in the third major zone, which runs obliquely to meet the iris-wreath at an angle of 30 deg. (injury sign—H). Diametrically opposite, at 60′ in the second major zone, another transversal begins at the iris-wreath and extends out to 5′ in the third major zone (J). This also indicates disturbance from injury, especially in view of the large divided dark sign enclosing the oblique transversal.

In view of the last two signs discussed, the possibility of earlier injury to the head should be investigated, remembering that such an injury could result in a disturbance of the medulla oblongata with consequent diabetes. In each of several cases of diabetes seen, no iris-sign for pancreatic involvement was visible, although an injury sign was present in the second and third major zones at 5′, thus confirming injury to the occiput.

However, from the large dark lacunae to be seen in this iris, hereditary predisposition to diabetes may be concluded, especially since similar large lacunae are also to be seen in the right iris. The injury may have been the precipitating cause for the onset of clinical symptoms.

The white clouds throughout the segments for neck and thorax, together with the dark signs and the heavy scurf-rim, which also appear in the right iris, suggest that tuberculosis must have affected the antecedents.

On the case record is noted: Housewife, 49 years of age, the seventh child of ten siblings, married with nine children. The father died from renal disease, the mother from heart failure. The paternal grandparents both lived to old age. The maternal grandfather died from senile weakness and the grandmother from pulmonary disease.

At 12 years of age the patient suffered from blood poisoning. At 18 years of age she fell from a haycart and broke the left lower leg, lying unconscious for two days. She had lived in very poor economic circumstances.

The patient presented at the first consultation with a suppurating ulcer of the upper right arm bone. During the subsequent three month period of treatment a very high reading for urinary sugar once again appeared, as well as pains in the ears with glandular swelling in the neck, which however completely resolved. During that period the patient had no further complaints until following some over-exertion an inflammation of the bone marrow in the right leg suddenly appeared. The urine sugar had risen to 7%. Since no improvement was apparent after treatment and the domestic circumstances required it, the patient had to be referred to hospital. After initial improvement of the leg condition, pneumonia developed, from which the patient died on the ninth day in hospital.

In view of the large heart signs in the iris, note the fatal issue of the pneumonia. The white flakes in the third major zone for the dorsal and thoracic areas are signs for catarrh of the lungs as affecting the entire thoracic organs and always signify a disposition to contract pneumonia.

Iris-37   **Female: 72 years—left iris**

Comparing this iris with Iris-36, it is immediately apparent that the large lacunae, which are such a prominent feature of the latter, are missing in Iris-37. This difference is based upon the relevant constitutional types:

Iris-36—nutritional type (pyknic), scrofulous constitution, disposed to catarrh of the mucous membranes.

Iris-37—sensitive type (leptosome), scrofulous constitution, disposed to nervous disturbances.

In contrast to Iris-36, the structure of Iris-37 is compact and only in the upper half are there some faintly indicated lacunae which may be assumed to be due to chronic cerebral circulatory insufficiency, leading to functional weakness of the central nervous system. The patient is lean, excitable and easily irritated.

Now consider the dark, closed lacuna at 12′ in the second major zone. It is a sign for a resolved cardiac condition, the probable consequence of an infectious disease contracted in youth. The small almost black elongated sign immediately above should be interpreted as a compensated valvular condition (A).

The two small closed signs at 19′ and 23′ in the third and fourth minor zones (B), together with the signs adjacent to the wreath at 40′, raise the question of pancreatic disturbance. The two small signs show conditions which have been resolved, although the small black points within the signs clearly indicate tissue damage involving the tail of the pancreas. External to the iris-wreath at 40′, and even more at 44′, the fibre structure is loosened and a white radial (inflammation-sign) is to be seen. Note also the fine black line which breaks through the iris-wreath to extend inwards as far as the first minor zone. This suggests that inflammatory adhesions between stomach and pancreas are present (C).

The apparent displacement upwards of the whole gastro-intestinal zone is significant and suggests that enlargement of an organ in the abdominal cavity has displaced stomach and intestine. The upwards displacement of the wreath is even more strongly apparent in the right iris, and a large black sign within the iris-wreath at 20′ has strong white clouds in the vicinity.

The case record states: The patient is a housewife, 72 years old, the youngest child of eight siblings, who were all diabetic. She is married and had two children. The father died when 60 years old from typhus. The mother died at the age of 75 years from senile weakness. No information is available concerning other relatives. The patient has been diabetic for seven years.

Three years before, a house-physician discovered an abdominal tumour the size of a walnut, but the finding was not confirmed in the clinic. After two and a half years, abdominal pains suddenly appeared which rendered the patient incapable of walking for a long time. Finally, a chance examination in Bad Neuenahr established the presence of a tumour in the stomach which was the size of the fist. The condition was treated initially with diathermy and then given two courses of ten deep-ray treatments without success. Operation was not possible. Further examination revealed a fist-size tumour in the regio-gastrica-dexter. The symptoms were a continuous diarrhoea and a sense of stomach pressure after eating rich foods. Several surgeons declined to operate. No further information is available concerning the ultimate outcome of the matter.

Iris-38   **Female: 69 years—left iris**

In this iris, the prominently white area at 10-16′ in the second major zone draws the attention and suggests calcification of the coronary vessels. The large, dark oval closed lacuna, almost enclosed by the white area, shows myocardial weakness, and the small elongated black sign close to the iris-wreath below signifies

111

myocardial damage, which must have been the consequence of infectious illness (A). The severe degree of coronary calcification probably arises from the gastro-intestinal disturbance, thus: gastro-intestinal dysfunction, pancreatic dysfunction, diabetes, general calcification, calcification of the coronary vessels.

The high blood pressure, which the patient has had for 10 years, arises from the heavy calcification of the entire vascular apparatus, in which the nervous system is also involved. The iris shows no evidence of renal disease.

Note the two black elongated signs at 20' and 22' in the second major zone (B). Both signs begin in the fourth minor zone. The lower of the two signs widens as it extends into the fifth minor zone. These two signs indicate pathology of the pancreas involving tissue degeneration, which is probably the reason for the excretion of sugar over the past fifteen years. However, since the signs lie further outwards in the fourth and fifth minor zones, it suggests that the condition is not severe and gives the patient no great trouble.

Observe the two small black signs at 41' at the iris-wreath and from which a dark wisp sign extends outwards to the iris-rim (C). This also refers to the pancreas and shows the long duration of the condition. The nutrition line (mouth-hand line) is also shown, for which the explanation given under Iris-36 is appropriate.

Note the transversals, which in this iris are so prominent. Beginning with the wavy line which commences at 35' at the iris-rim, extends upwards through the fourth minor zone to end at the iris-wreath at 43' (D), this sign indicates injury to the back which has produced a spinal distortion. In relation to this, note the transversal which begins at 46' in the wreath and extends to the iris-rim at 54' (E), and the fine white line in the shoulder area from 7' to 14' (F). These lines are signs of injury, which was probably sustained in a fall from a swing (see case history).

The long black sign at 26', which begins at a sharp indentation of the iris-wreath and extends outwards to the small white cross lines (cobweb sign) which cover the area of the third major zone between 23' and 30', representing the peritoneum, is a defect sign. This sign is the probable result of a suppurative focus in the left abdomen. The possible cause is a perforation of the intestine. Cobweb signs indicate adhesions (agglutinations) which arise from inflammation of the serous membranes. This patient's childlessness is likely to be due to obstruction of the Fallopian tubes from adhesions.

The patient is a small, gentle creature, and leads a moderate way of life. She needs neither insulin, nor a special diet. The urine sugar level maintains at 1-3%. The high blood pressure varied during a long period of treatment between 170mm. and 240mm. The patient died at the age of 81 years. The immediate cause of death is not known.

The case record gives the following details: The patient is a housewife, 69 years of age, the third child of seven siblings. She was married, but had no children. The patient's father died at 77 years of age from bronchial catarrh. The mother died at 49 years of age with Bright's disease. Of the six brothers and sisters of the mother, one brother died at the age of 50 years from diabetes. One son of another brother is similarly diabetic.

Earlier illness: The patient contracted all the usual childhood diseases. At the age of 12 years, she fell from a swing and was ill for a long time. At the age of 18 years she lay for six months in spinal traction on account of spinal curvature. A reading for urine-sugar has been present for 15 years and the blood pressure was found to be high 10 years ago. The symptoms at the first consultation were: stomach pressure, eructations and constipation.

Iris-39   **Female: 52 years—left iris**

Considering the iris generally, an immediate impact is made by the large dark lacunae which cover almost the entire surface. Similar lacunae are even more prominent in the right iris, thus indicating hereditary weaknesses.

This iris has very many similarities to Iris-36, and the patients are similar in appearance. The white catarrh signs so strongly evident in Iris-36 are not so clearly shown here. However, they appear more prominent in the right iris, again confirming the hereditary disposition. The patient weighs 170 lbs. and is only 160 cms. in height.

The large first major zone, which is wider towards the temporal side, indicates over-relaxation of the intestinal musculature. The large, dark sign at 15′ in the second and third major zone, which extends to the sixth minor zone, shows myocardial weakness. The fact that the position of this sign is relatively low, is probably consistent with a general displacement of all signs due to bodily distortion and weakening of the internal organs (ptosis) following injury to the left shoulder. This involves rigidity of the neck and a deviation of the head towards the left. The sign indicates gross myocardial weakness with dilatation, the latter suggested by the considerable widening in the fourth minor zone (A).

Observe the long open lacuna at 40', where the iris-wreath deviates strongly towards the pupillary margin (B). The sign refers to the pancreas and involves adhesion to the posterior wall of the stomach resulting from inflammation. This constitutes a considerable stress for the organism, especially in view of the downward strain from the general visceroptosis.

In the spring of 1939, acute inflammation of the pancreas developed, which was treated as gastric catarrh. The condition did not improve, the patient's weight declined from 170 lbs. to 135 lbs. and there was thirst and abdominal irritation. Observing the area at 20', adjacent to the iris-wreath, no special sign is visible, other than a small white cloud in the intensely white area close to the wreath, showing that inflammation has affected the islet apparatus.

The closed dark lacuna at 33' in the second major zone is a sign for weakness of the renal function (C). The lower position of the sign also suggests ptosis, although there is not a floating kidney, as described for Iris-18. In this case, it is more a question of stasis, in which the ptosis is probably no more than a few centimetres. The stasis of urine in the kidney is likely to arise from the pressure of a left ovarian tumour, indicated by the large, dark sign at 25-28' in the second and third major zones. In fact, there are two signs, which are separated by no more than a fine, thin arc-line (D).

The sign adjacent to the iris-wreath indicates vascular stasis in the pelvic basin, whereas the wide, dark sign towards the periphery represents the tumour of the left ovary. Note the border of the ovary sign (swelling) in the arc-line to the leg area. These signs together with the heart signs, provide the explanation for the dark sign at 30-33' (E), showing that swelling and stasis of the leg arises on the one hand from the ovarian tumour and on the other, from the myocardial weakness.

The suprarenal sign is still to be discussed. This is the small, dark sign at 30' between the ovary sign and the kidney sign, adjacent to the iris-wreath (F). If, as in this case, a kidney sign is seen in the left iris, a tuberculous disposition should be considered. If there is also a suprarenal sign, suggesting autonomic disturbance, then proceed very carefully. Since both signs press in towards the pupil, digestive disturbance is also indicated.

The four closed lacunae lying one under the other between 42′ and 50′ in the second major zone have the same explanation as that given for Iris-36. The large, open lacuna at 3′ in the second and third major zones, diametrically opposite the kidney sign, illustrates the relationship between the renal function and the midbrain. It is not without significance that renal hypertension affects visual power so strongly.

The large lacuna in the area for cerebrum, extended still further by the closed lacuna lying diametrically opposite the pancreas sign at 38′, shows the effect of dysfunction in the organs of metabolism. This produces disorder in the muscular and circulatory apparatus, which in turn results in a collapse of the hormone system and ultimate decline in mento-emotional capacity. Consequently, such patients are stupid and taciturn (G).

The following notes appear on the case record: The patient is a housewife, 52 years of age, the tenth child of twelve siblings, married with two children. The father died at 70 years of age from a cerebral haemorrhage. The mother died at the age of 69 years when she had been ill for only three days.

Earlier illnesses: As a child the patient had many colds. She had measles. A perineal laceration was sustained during the first childbirth. Following a decline in body weight from 170 lbs. to 135 lbs., the doctor examined the urine periodically over a period of eighteen months, but without result. The patient once fell on the left side and broke the arm and ribs. There is now a distorted posture of the head towards the left side.

At the first consultation, the patient presented with the following symptoms: abdominal irritation, rheumatic conditions, left sciatic pain, considerable swelling of the left leg in the evening. The urine gave a positive reading for sugar content.

Irides 36-39 represent four patients with diabetes, in which the condition is discussed in relation to other signs in the second major zone (blood and muscle rings). It is evident that the signs are not uniform in the different patients.

When diabetes develops as the result of a disturbance in the medulla oblongata, iris signs of injury may be found in the area for cerebellum if an accident was the cause of the disturbance.

Moreover, the case history will often show that diabetes appears following conditions affecting the lungs and kidneys or from hereditary consequences.

Iris-40   **Female: 62 years—right iris**

On initial examination of this iris, attention is immediately arrested by the large, black sign at 43-48′ (A). Similar signs are found in the right iris where there are hereditary influences of bronchial disease (asthma), or where severe whooping cough was contracted during childhood. The small black signs at 12′ in the second major zone, with the oblique pattern of black signs lying one under the other in the third major zone, indicate pharyngeal catarrh (B). In relation to these signs, note the statements on the case records.

Consideration of the first major zone in the lower sector between 20′ and 40′ shows a markedly zig-zag form of the iris-wreath and a generally upward displacement. From these signs it may be deduced that the organs of the second major zone have been the subject of repeated inflammatory activity which has implicated the contiguous intestinal structures. It has recently been observed that where there is acute inflammation of the kidney, the typical white cloud extended as far as the intestinal area. When the inflammation receded, the iris-wreath in that sector remained indented towards the pupil.

To understand the extent of the severe and chronic condition present in this patient, the signs in the second major zone between 22′ and 40′ must be considered together. It can be seen that this whole area is surrounded by a white zig-zag line (C). Beginning at 21′ at the iris-wreath and following the white line almost to the outer iris-rim at 26′, the area for bladder is demarcated towards the back. From 26′ the white line extends obliquely to the outer limit of the second major zone at 30′. This outward deviation, together with the white wisp sign at 25′, shows inflammation of the urethra and burning of the vagina, arising from the purulent state of the urine. From 30′ the white line proceeds outwards to the leg area at 32′, where pelvic visceral adhesions have developed from inflammation of the ureters. The line then extends through an area of small white flakes and streaks to 37′, showing the extent of peritoneal adhesions involving the appendix and the small intestine. From 37′, a thicker, oblique line proceeds to 40′, from which point several branches extend to the iris-wreath.

Here at 40′, inside the iris-wreath, the descending part of the duodenum has its location. From the signs described, it is evident that adhesions have resulted from chronic inflammatory irritation and although the causative renal condition produces many symptoms, yet the most severe pains will arise from the duodenal involvement, which is to be assessed as a secondary disturbance. The white zig-zag line, beginning close to the pupil at 37′ and extending out to the periphery, is a special indicator for pain on this side of the abdomen (D).

A note concerning 'stone-signs': When concretions form in a hollow organ, there will be no sign in the iris for so long as the surrounding tissues are not affected. If, for example, concretions exist in the renal pelvis which irritate the mucous membrane and stimulate an inflammatory reaction, a white colouring will be seen in the kidney area of the iris. The greater the inflammatory response, the more extensive is the white colouring. However, if erosion of tissue occurs from the same cause, then a black sign develops in the corresponding area. In this iris, small black signs denoting tissue damage can be seen. The small and large white areas and points show inflammation. Since everything has been affected by the scar tissue adhesions, it is not possible to differentiate individual organs.

The case record notes the following details: The patient is a housewife, 62 years of age, married with ten children. The father died from pneumonia. The mother died from senile weakness at the age of 96 years. The two brothers of the father suffered from asthma and the paternal grandfather also had asthma. The paternal grandmother died in childbirth.

Earlier illnesses: The patient suffered from milk-scurf as an infant and developed severe whooping cough during childhood. During childbirth at the age of 25 years, a renal haemorrhage occurred, and two years later stones as large as hen's eggs were found in both kidneys.

The symptoms and conditions recorded at the first consultation were: headache, stomach pressure, nausea, vomiting, constipation. For a long time the patient suffered from cough with expectoration, irritation and burning of the anus and vagina, frequent colicky pains in the right abdomen and ureteral colic. The urine was highly purulent.

Iris-41/42   **Male: 33 years—left/right iris**

Iris-41, the left iris, shows a prominent closed lacuna in the heart area, at 13′ in the second major zone. The sign probably appeared in youth following diphtheria and being closed, shows that the condition is no longer active. Detailed examination shows a small black sign under the upper white border of the lacuna and towards the pupil and a larger black sign further outwards. These signs should be regarded as indicating valvular lesions which have been compensated. The loosening of the radial fibres around the lacuna reflects the condition which now exists (A).

If in the presence of such a valve defect decompensation for some reason occurs, then the condition would be serious and other signs are looked for, as may be seen here. Since the entire heart sign extends from 10′ to 18′ and out into the third major zone, considerable enlargement is likely and the existence of long black signs between the thick white lines shows that atrophic changes affect the myocardium (B).

Now consider the dark sign at 42-45′ in the second major zone, diametrically opposite the closed heart sign (C). It will be seen that here also there are black signs between the white lines. This suggests that the enlarged heart is causing pressure upon the tissues lying posteriorly, with consequent damage to the spinal column. This sign similarly indicates the gravity of the patient's conditition and no further improvement can be promised.

The large open lacuna with the thick white border, immediately above the sign last discussed at 45-50′ in the second and third major zones, actually consists of three lacunae and signifies catarrh of the throat with involvement of the oesophagus (D). This sign can be properly assessed only if considered together with the white flakes at 15′ and the dark to black signs in the lung area at 10-18′ in the third major zone. These signs show catarrhal states of the air passages with expectoration, the latter condition seen in the open back sign below the large white flake and the white tufts extending outwards from the white cloud to the iris-rim (E). These signs should be related to those in the throat area. The two black points

118

within the black line at 48' in the third major zone are generally found following diphtheria.

The white bordered sign at 30-38' in the second and third major zones, enclosing an area of loose texture, suggests kidney disease (F). A cystic and suppurative condition of the kidney on the left with renal stasis from ureteral obstruction on the right is bound to produce a cardiac stress. From the consequent stasis in the pulmonary circulation a catarrhal state of the bronchi has developed which can lead to asthmatic conditions.

To the kidney signs: Note the heavy white line as an arc at 37' in the second and third major zones, showing inflammation of the kidney and the surrounding tissues. However, the inner border to the long, black sign is rather straight. This thick, straight line, together with the somewhat oblique, thick, short white line going from 31' to 34' in the second major zone, as far as the iris-wreath, indicates that the kidney has been affected by an injury, the long black sign suggesting tissue destruction. The small, black sign extending obliquely from the latter to 30' in the third major zone, also shows tissue destruction with suppuration (F).

The long subdivided black sign at 29-30' is not part of the kidney sign but refers to the leg area. The sign does not begin at the iris-wreath as does the kidney sign, but extends outwards from the fourth into the fifth minor zone. The sign has arisen from the severe suppurative condition of the left knee joint. Note the small transversals to be seen within and below the sign, showing that the cause was an injury (G).

Right iris (Iris-42)-

As already stated, there is a condition of hydronephrosis affecting the right kidney, in which stasis is caused by obstruction of the ureter. Consider first the group of small black signs beginning at 7' in the third major zone (frontal sinus) and extending as an almost vertical line down to the neck area at 15' in the third major zone (H). These signs show that a suppurative infection of the frontal sinus has involved the whole naso-pharyngeal cavity in inflammation and degeneration of the mucous membrane, as well as the teeth.

The large, dark sign in this same area adjacent to the iris-wreath shows catarrh of the air-passages (J). Diametrically opposite to this sign at 44', black signs are seen between the white clouds in the second and third major zones (K), showing catarrh of the bronchi with degeneration of the mucous membrane. Adhesions are also present, originating from an old pleural inflammation.

The white coloured clouds are, in fact, not quite snow-white but tend towards a grey-white, indicating that the inflammatory process affecting the mucous membrane has reached a chronic stage. Compare with the signs for the same areas in the left iris and the descriptions given.

The dark, open lacuna with a wide, white border at 28' in the second major zone, is a sign for inflammation and enlargement of the kidney (L). Within the lacuna, small dark points are present which indicate weakened, but not yet destroyed, tissues. However, the dark signs below this lacuna, which extend as an expansion towards 30', confirm the destructive tendencies (M).

The dark open lacuna at 24-25' in the second major zone is a sign for weakness of the bladder, in which the small black points indicate degeneration of the mucous membrane (N). If adhesions affecting the ureter have been already established, the appropriate signs should be looked for at 32-35'. The white colouring here shows inflammation affecting the lower right abdominal organs, and the small lines indicate adhesions arising from injury.

The dark sign at 33-35' in the fifth minor zone suggests involvement of the right testicle, and the small, black point at 34' at the iris-wreath implies participation of the intestine with local ulceration due to the adhesions. (P) That the process is now resolved is shown by the white surrounding border to the sign. It is indeed possible that the intestinal ulceration affecting the caecal area has been responsible for the adhesion pathology in the whole region, as anyone knowing the anatomical relations within the lower abdomen would agree.

The black sign commencing at 38' in the iris-wreath, in which the peak lies in the second minor zone and the sign extends through the wreath to the periphery, shows the effect upon the gall-bladder and liver of a disturbance originating in the duodenum (R). The low position of the sign is consistent with the general visceroptosis suggested by the widened ventral section of the first major zone. Only the kidney and bladder signs displace the wreath inwards. Indeed, it is because of the gastro-intestinal conditions that the consequences of the injury have been so severe.

Assuming that the dark area from 55' to 5' in the right iris existed before the cerebral concussion following the motor-cycle

120

accident, then it is not surprising that such an incident occurred. A large area of darker colour in this sector of the iris, diametrically opposite the bright white colouring in the lower quadrant, strongly suggests that there was a state of cerebral ischaemia. Appearing, as it does, in the right iris indicates the probability of hereditary encumbrance.

The following details are noted on the case record: The patient was a bricklayer, 33 years of age, married with one child. The earlier illnesses were: measles and diphtheria during childhood. When 15 years old he fell from a building, injuring his left side with a coffee-flask in the left pocket. The kidney disturbance commenced subsequently, although the condition was not at first taken seriously. Three years later, a motor-cycle accident resulted in concussion and an injury to the left knee, which developed cell-tissue inflammation and suppuration, needing to be lanced several times. At 18 years of age he developed inflammation of the right lung and pleura. At 25 years of age all teeth were extracted because of paradontosis and root abscesses. In October 1938 the patient was in Bad Wildungen, where radiographs of the kidneys were taken. Because of the presence of adhesions the right kidney could not be filled. The left kidney was filled and showed the presence of a cystic condition which it was assumed would become larger. The patient died in January 1939.

Iris-43/44   **Female: 32 years—right/left iris**

The iris photographs are those of a young woman, for whom the case record states as follows: The patient is the fourth of five children, is now married and has one child. The father at 62 years of age and the mother at 61 years of age are both in good health.

The patient is small and asthenic with bright red-blonde hair and domed finger-nails. The little finger is sharply bent outwards at the middle joint, a feature which is not present in the other children. The small mouth is striking and the nose is strongly inclined. The iris is grey-blue. Of the brothers and sisters, two have dark brown irides. During infancy the patient had pleurisy with suppurative effusion. At six years of age, inflammation of the middle ear developed which was unrecognised. Active tuberculosis was discovered when the patient was 29 years old.

121

The patient came for her first consultation on 18.1.39, having previously undertaken three courses of treatment in a sanatorium. The examination findings were: height 1.58 m., weight 54 kg., symptoms of huskiness, cough with expectoration, night sweats, loss of appetite, pains in the right ribs and sticking pain in the back, suppurating ears, frequent but scanty micturition. She discharged herself from the sanatorium on 20.12.38 as not cured. Pneumothorax could not be applied, thoracoplasty was suggested but not carried out.

Intensive homoeopathic treatment produced good results, so that by 14.6.39 there were no further night sweats or cough and the appetite had improved. The weight was 53 kg. The patient presented herself again on 25.1.40 and had remained in good health. In May 1940 she was once again sent for a course of treatment, since a cavity had again broken down following a contagious cold. In October 1940, she reported having been discharged as completely cured. Her weight was then 50 kg.

In January 1941 the patient attended again for consultation. She felt well and the weight had recovered to 52.5 kg. Unfortunately, for technical reasons, it was not possible to repeat the iris photographs. The photographs shown were those made at the first consultation. The patient has not been seen since.

To the iris signs: The large white stomach ring in both irides shows chronic catarrh of the stomach with increased acid formation. The peaked dilatations of the intestinal ring also suggest chronic catarrh with colic. From 36′ to 43′ in the first major zone of the right iris, small, elongated black signs are shown which at 40′ project as a long spike into the second major zone (A). These are signs for adhesions following ulceration of the pylorus and duodenum.

The small dark lacuna at 35′ in the second major zone, adjacent to the large spike, relates to the pancreas (B). This is involved with the adhesions to the duodenum, as are the black signs in the large spike at 49-50′ (C). That part of the large intestine before the hepatic flexure also participates. There is here a hereditary condition which is very much affected by the general state of health.

The large lacunae in the areas for the respiratory organs (bronchi and lungs at 42-52′, trachea at 12-15′ in the second major zone) are especially prominent. Since the signs are so large, extending into the third major zone, and also cover the shoulder area, it is evident that the skeletal system is involved (D).

The large area of dark colouring at 17-22′ also implies weakness, so that too much exertion should not be required of the patient. Since these signs are especially prominent in the right eye, a hereditary predisposition is implied (E). Moreover, patients with such signs are themselves unable to judge the degree of weakness present and always over-exert themselves.

Consider the large dark sign at 28-32′ (F). Since this kidney sign extends so far, a condition of stasis and swelling is suggested, and the displacement towards 32′ raises the question of a possible floating kidney.

The suprarenal sign at 33′, adjacent to the iris-wreath (G), lies diametrically opposite the pituitary sign at 2′ (H), showing disturbance of endocrine functions. At 3′ in the fourth and fifth minor zones, there is a sign showing one-half quite dark and the other half containing white fibres (J). This sign indicates disturbance of the forebrain and should be considered together with ovarian dysfunction shown by the white sign at 33′ and the long white lines at 35′ (K).

The large, dark sign at 55′, which is closed towards 53′, shows disturbance of the cerebellum (L). Since the iris-wreath is strongly contracted in this sector, involvement of the vegetative nervous system is indicated.

A continuous inflammatory process is shown by the white clouds in the sixth minor zone, particularly implicating the frontal sinus, throat and mouth (7-13′), dorsal pleura (16-21′), and lungs (45-50′).

The open lacunae between 42′ and 50′ suggest that destructive processes are still active and especially involving the lungs. The two small black signs at 48′ and 49′ indicate cavitation of the upper and middle lobes (M).

Left iris—

Large lacunae are also to be seen in the second and third major zones of the left iris, covering the areas for mouth, neck and back, and showing all signs open. Thus, the disturbance is still active and there is an acute condition of weakness. The large sign at 46-50′ suggests catarrh of the throat and larynx with expectoration (N). The oesophagus is also involved. A long dark sign between white radial lines at 18′ in the sector for upper extremity (P) emphasises the hand-mouth line (nutrition line) and implies that conditions arise from faulty diet. Also, secondary infection from the swallowing of bacilli-containing sputum involves the tissues of the oesophagus and stomach.

The closed lacuna at 32′ is a sign for an earlier renal pathology (R). The white border at the upper part of the sign towards the iris-wreath suggests existing inflammation.

The closed suprarenal sign at 29′ indicates autonomic stress (S), also confirmed by the narrowing of the wreath opposite the signs for kidney and suprarenal gland. As in the right iris, there is a sign for the pituitary body (T) diametrically opposite to that for the suprarenal gland and signs showing the connection of forebrain (55′) and ovary (25-28′).

An acute myocardial weakness is shown by the small open signs in the heart area at 12-17′. The dark sign at 16′ shows a tendency to dropsical swelling (V). In relation to this, the dark sign at 29-32′ in the fourth to sixth minor zones is appropriate for oedematous swelling of the left leg.

As in the right iris, so here the white flakes refer to the same organs and have the same interpretation. Where the white flakes and white radials extend outwards to the iris-rim, skin eruptions are indicated. In the right iris, the destructive sign for the lung area is from 47′ to 50′, whereas in the left iris the open lacunae are seen in the dorsal areas between 40′ and 50′. Even though the iris fibres in this area are loosened, cavitation is not established with certainty.

The web-signs in the rib and lung areas showing adhesions, the haemorrhoid sign in the area for rectum and the injury sign in the leg area should be noted. Although the patient was at first discharged as cured, yet the state of encumbrance affecting all organs is so grave that a fresh outbreak of the disease is always to be expected.

The following clinical indications are all very bad signs:
Small mouth = insufficient food intake.
Strong growth of hair = severe deprivation of silicic acid.
Red-blonde hair = sensitive organism, especially to sunlight.
High-domed finger nails = renal disturbance.

Comparing these irides with 43 and 44, it is apparent that irides 45 and 46 are almost completely covered with grey-white deposits, whereas in the preceding pictures the lower layers are visible (second layer = vascular) and surface deposits are almost completely absent. This is probably to be explained by the considerable difference in the state of the lymphatic system in the individual constitutions—

Iris-43/44: there is too little fluid in the tissues with general emaciation, even though oedematous swelling of the feet exists. (Left iris: suprarenal sign shows tendency to emaciation and vegetative dystony.)

Iris-45/46: there is too much fluid in the tissues, bloated corpulency with general and facial swelling but no oedema of the feet. The eyes are especially affected since the kidneys are severely diseased.

However, it will not be sufficient to look for the cause solely in terms of cardiac and renal conditions, even if these can be established as hereditary tendencies, but to include other predisposing factors. In addition, the relevant constitution should be assessed, since this is not solely a matter of heredity. In my opinion, constitution is the summation of hereditary predisposition together with nutritional and environmental conditioning.

Irides 45 and 46 show many dark-brown flecks which will appear on the monochrome photographs as black deposits. These indications are not to be confused with true black signs (defect-signs) which arise from the dissolution of the surface tissues and are to be seen as deep holes. Comparing the right with the left iris, it is noticeable that the former is more extensively covered with white clouds (hereditary disposition).

Right iris—

The outer edge of the first minor zone is too white, showing inflammation of the muscular layer of the stomach. The state of the inner margin (pupillary) shows coarseness of the mucosal folds with deterioration of the mucous membrane. The second minor zone is only visible between 32' and 52' and has many small black signs, indicating chronic intestinal catarrh with mucosal degeneration.

At 35' in the first minor zone, close observation shows two black signs with white borders, of which one sign begins open at the pupillary margin (gastric ulcer). The closed black sign adjacent to it in the intestinal zone shows a resolved condition. This sign lies in the caecal area and the suspended black sign indicates disease of the appendix (A).

At 40-42' in the first and second minor zones, a white oblique line is seen in an area of general fibre looseness. These are signs for inflammation and ulceration affecting the pylorus and duodenum (B). The small intestine area at 5-33' shows dilatations with signs for tissue degeneration. These indications are less prominent. The black deposits at 15' in the first major zone, together with those in the second major zone at 15', 28-30', 33-38' and 54', are toxin-signs.

The black sign in the throat area at 13-15' in the third major zone shows mucous membrane deterioration (C). The large black signs in the lung area, 44-51', and more especially at 44-47', show that destructive processes are active in the lung tissue. The white arc-line at 44', which extends from the iris-wreath to the periphery, shows swelling and exudation with inflammation of the serous membrane (D).

At 37', a thick white line extends from the iris-wreath almost to the iris-rim and a white zig-zag line ascends obliquely to meet the white arc at 44'. This suggests that the inflammation has encroached upon the diaphragm (E). From 37' to 50' in the sixth minor zone there are cobweb-signs and between 17' and 25' the thick transversals show adhesions.

The kidney sign at 27-33', reaching from the iris-wreath out into the third major zone, shows loosening of the radial fibres with destructive indications. The wide extent of the sign suggests swelling and displacement, and the thick white arc bordering the sign shows inflammation affecting the contiguous tissues (F).

Left iris—

The signs in the first major zone of the left iris are worse than those in the right iris. The seeming upward displacement of the whole zone is due to abdominal distension, probably arising from the state of the kidneys and bladder.

The very wide kidney sign, spanning 24-34', indicates hydronephrosis with displacement (cystic kidney) (G). Likewise, the wide bladder sign containing black defect-signs shows swelling with tissue degeneration (H).

Many black defect-signs may be seen in the segment 20-25′, abdominal cavity, which refer to destruction of the lymph nodes (J). Although the pulmonary sectors in this iris are less prominent, there are signs of tissue destruction to be seen. This iris emphasises the considerable pathology affecting the kidney and bladder and the abdominal organs generally.

Case record—

The patient is a joiner, 29 years of age, single, with two brothers/sisters. The father is 55 years of age and still living. The mother died from tuberculosis at 28 years of age. No information is recorded concerning other ancestors.

As a child the patient contracted measles and pneumonia. At 12 years of age he was ill for a long time and for one year had inflammation of the renal pelvis. Four weeks previously he was in hospital for three days to undertake a water cure. Urination was induced by irrigation of the bladder.

At the second consultation the patient complained of stomach pressure, diarrhoea and haemorrhoids, apart from the pain in the back and bladder. After four treatments he was referred for further in-patient treatment. The patient died from renal tuberculosis.

Iris-47/48   **Female: 28 years—right/left iris**

On comparing these pictures with the others in the series, the coarse structure of the iris-fibres is immediately obvious. This type of structure is described as 'combed-hair' (after Maubach) and regarded by many as suggesting a cancerous state. However, this is only so provisionally. The fact that this structure is so frequently found in cancer patients is to be taken as indicating no more than the decline of vital powers characteristic of every wasting disease in the advanced stages.

According to my interpretation, anyone may develop tuberculosis but does not need to. The same applies to cancer. That it can be so lies in the hereditary tendencies, the environmental influences, and above all in the nutrition. In this case, I will explain the most important signs in relation to each other and conclude by quoting the entries on the case record.

In the right iris, with its almost square-shaped first major zone, a severe condition of gastro-intestinal catarrh may be deduced from the mixture of black and white signs. Ignoring other considerations, the square-shaped wreath together with the peaked expansions of the wreath along the ear-bladder line provide a grave prognosis, as well as indicating hereditary weakness of those organs (A). A similar large expansion at 16' in the dorsal area, together with the long black sign at 18' in the second major zone, indicate stress affecting the back (B).

The long black sign at 11' and 12' in the second and third major zones indicates chronic catarrh of the pharynx and bronchi (C). The pronounced loosening of the radial fibres at 43' to 47' in the lung area likewise shows chronic catarrh (D).

The large dark sign at 54-56', showing similar loosening of the radial structure, indicates insufficient circulation to the brain (E). This may be explained by the sign for inflammation and acute activity in the area for uterus and vagina at 24-27'. Inflammation and over-activity in the lower abdomen (white signs) leads to circulatory insufficiency in the head. However, the long black signs in the same area show degeneration of the mucous membranes (F).

The first major zone is not so square-shaped in the left iris as in the right. However, both the black and white signs and the sharply notched expansions of the iris-wreath reveal the severe state of gastro-intestinal catarrh and the basis of the strong colicky pains.

The two black signs at 35' in the area for rectum, together with the large intestinal spike at 25', show a severe condition of the colon which extends to the anus (G). The adjacent thick white sign at 36' is to be interpreted as an acute inflammatory sign for the rectum. Together with the large white cloud at 37' next to the iris-wreath and the small black signs at 37' in the third major zone, the signs also show inflammation of the bladder and urethra (H).

The white constriction sign at 31', which extends inwards as far as the pupillary margin, together with a similar sign in the right iris at 29', indicate chronic renal inflammation affecting both kidneys which has already existed for a long time (J).

The black sign at 13' adjacent to the area of loose radial structure within the heart sign (13-16'), appears as though it might lie inside the iris-wreath. This wedge sign in the second major zone should be regarded as very serious (K).

The loose radial fibre structure is also apparent in the lung area (10-17'), as also in the cranial area at 60-7', which lies opposite the signs for over-activity in the area for lower abdomen and rectum. From the white deposits (flakes) in the sixth minor zone, a generalised acute state of the mucous membranes may be presumed, and since these signs extend out to the iris-rim, the existence of skin eruption and exudations is likely.

Notes on the case record:
Female patient, 28 years of age, ladies help, the ninth child of eleven siblings, two of which died from diphtheria.

Father 68 years of age, mother 63 years of age, both healthy and blue eyed.

The patient has a lymphatic constitution, blue eyes, dark blonde hair, clubbed fingers, thin face with a red hectic flush on the cheeks, thick nose, unclean skin with pustules and ulcers on the face.

The patient had diphtheria at the age of 5 years, influenza at the age of 15 years and pleurisy at the age of 20 years. Since puberty severe disturbances related to the period. For three years she has been treated by the doctor for bronchial catarrh, had the lungs radiographed but no abnormality was found.

At the first consultation the following complaints were recorded—Morning and evening cough, especially with changes of temperature. For the past eight weeks has suffered pains in the stomach with vomiting. Belching eased the symptoms. Total chronic constipation. Pain on micturition, so delay in emptying the bladder. Otherwise, few occasions of passing water. Scalp irritation, wet discharge behind the ears and ulcers on the face. Haemorrhoids with anal irritation. Strong vaginal discharge with burning and irritation. There has been no menstrual period for the past seven weeks.

Clinical findings:
Heart muscle weakness, cardiac neurosis, hereditary cardiac condition. Catarrh of the apices of the lungs, bronchial catarrh with coarse rales everywhere. Abdomen distended and everywhere painful on pressure. Urine contains albumin and pus. Weight 49 Kg.

Treatment: Tuberculosis remedies prescribed together with other medicines for stomach, intestines, kidneys, bladder, etc., according to the variable symptoms.

The patient died from abdominal tuberculosis.

At the first consultation the iris indications of a tubercular background were quite distinct. By this example I wished to show how important is the diagnosis from the iris for recognition of the basic origin of an illness.

Iris-49/50   **Female: 39 years—right/left iris**

The patient is 39 years of age, single, a seamstress, the first child of four siblings, sensitive type. The fingernails had transverse grooves, the skin was delicate with a rose-coloured complexion, the face was long and thin. During childhood the patient contracted measles. Later she was treated for many years for conditions of the liver and gall-bladder. In March, 1938, tuberculosis was discovered with cavitation in the right lung and treated ambulantly.

At the first consultation on 16.6.1939 she complained of pain in the region of the left kidney, a purulent discharge and burning on micturition, a cough with heavy green expectoration, heart pains and stitches. On 6.7.1939, the patient attended again when the findings were worse than before.

The parents of the patient were both still alive and healthy. Of the three brothers/sisters of the father, one sister had died from kidney disease. Of the four brothers/sisters of the mother, one sister with abdominal cancer had died at operation. The father's parents had lived to old age. The mother's parents: the mother was still alive at 80 years of age but no information was available concerning the father.

In this case, were a good heredity to be assumed, then it would follow that the conditions would be due to an encumbrance of the organism arising from insufficient elimination through the kidneys and skin. Since, however, of the antecedents one sister of the father died at 50 years of age with kidney disease and one sister of the mother with abdominal cancer, then it must be taken that the heredity is poor, even though the parents are apparently healthy. The earlier liver and gall-bladder conditions are probably the result of faulty nutrition. Even though the profession of seamstress, alone in a large city, does not exactly provide the best possible nutrition, yet there are many in similar conditions who remain healthy and have no tuberculosis.

Considering the iris in general, the first and second major zones are too light, whereas the peripheral region covering the third major zone and the scurf rim is too dark. This arises from insufficient elimination through the skin. In addition, there are many reddish-yellow deposits distributed over the first and second major zones, representing intoxications which produce general encumbrance of the nervous system.

Right iris—

Apart from the general depositions, there is a line of white flakes in the third major zone between 13' and 37', which signify chronic catarrh or irritation of the serous membranes. A shorter series is seen at 42-48'. The fact that the signs lie so far inwards at 15' and 45' and that from 13' the line of flakes proceeds almost vertically down to 27' is of grave significance (A). The inward position implies that no elimination through the skin at that level is possible, but since the signs extend downwards and outwards as far as the lower abdomen, then it is evident that the same condition affects the lower tissues and that elimination will take place there. Even if some elimination takes place through the bronchi (signs at 13'), yet the mucous membranes of the nose and frontal sinus do not participate. The large, dark sign in the second and third major zone at 13-15' shows severe catarrh of the trachea with some atrophic degeneration (small long dark signs within the large lacuna) (B).

Observe the long, dark sign at 43' and 44' (C). This indicates a severe condition of the bronchi. The pattern of sign-structure seen here, in fact extends to cover the whole area of the lungs (44-50'), and signifies a gradual destruction of the tissues as may be seen in the last stages of all serious pathology, including cancer. There are no special signs for disease names and even where there are large cavities, the form of the corresponding sign needs a practised eye to elucidate.

The looser iris-texture in the sector 37-39' results from earlier liver and gall-bladder disease. The three white zig-zag lines which extend to the iris-rim show that the condition is still present and that painful symptoms will follow dietetic indiscretions (D).

At 37' in the second major zone, the white lines include segments of arc and there is a half-moon shaped dark sign (E). This formation suggests the existence of a tumour, in this case, a distended gall-bladder.

The darkened area between 23' and 27' in the second and third major zones becomes even darker as it extends towards the periphery. This suggests catarrh of the bladder and uterus with discharge (F).

Left iris—
In the left iris, the large dark sign at 30-33′ refers to the kidney. Such signs in the left iris give a general indication of tuberculosis (G). The textural looseness in the iris is less apparent than in the right, but there are increased white and coloured deposits. The inward displacement of the white flakes in the dorsal area between 30′ and 50′, whereby the dark scurf-rim is markedly widened, indicates severe encumbrance.

The dark signs between 17′ and 27′ in the second and third major zones which on close observation look faintly like lacunae, together with the loosening of the radial fibres at 10-17′, 40-45′ and 50-56′, suggest a general weakness of structures within the abdominal cavity, especially affecting the muscular elements (H).

However, the real dissolution and destruction takes place in the respiratory organs. Since the whole of the lung tissue is involved, there are no special signs for cavitation, and in this patient, even with the best of means, no further improvement can be obtained.

Iris-51/52   **Male: right/left iris**

These irides differ from those of the preceding six patients in their basic structure. Persons with such compact and finely textured irides have a very sensitive nervous system and are otherwise highly reactive. According to quite recent observations, this does not depend upon hereditary factors alone, but also involves the considerable influence of nutrition and environment. From insufficient cellulose, over-concentrated foods and high fat intake, disturbance of the stomach is produced which extends to the duodenum and in turn results in stasis of liver and pancreas.

Note the signs at 38′ and 40′ in the first to third major zones of the right iris. Light colouring together with dark to black signs are seen covering the areas from pylorus to the liver (A). The excessive consumption of carbohydrate in the form of white sugar, white bread and cakes, produces gastro-intestinal disturbance. From the lack of saliva (insufficient mastication) and pancreatic secretion (obstruction of the pancreatic duct) the conversion of carbohydrate to grape sugar is prevented, or at least greatly disturbed.

Fermentation of the unreduced carbohydrate irritates the intestinal mucosa. This, and the lack of cellulose, induces over-contraction of the intestine. Note the large stomach ring and the small intestinal ring.

Lack of cellulose in the nutrition renders the function of the appendix superfluous and the organ declines. Note the signs at 33-35' in the intestinal area of the right iris (caecal area). Small black points are to be seen at this location, as well as a large white cloud in the third major zone (B). (The photograph was taken 14 days after an operation on the appendix and there were still pains in the caecal region).

That the faulty nutrition also affects the rectum is shown by the signs at 34-36' in the third major zone of the left iris, representing haemorrhoids and inflammation of the mucous membrane (C). The small black signs over the whole of the area for large intestine between 60' and 30' are defect-signs, showing a condition of chronic catarrh with local defects of the mucous membrane. The iris shows here the effects of pathological contraction, with stasis and anal inflammation.

The reader may now wonder why these irides should be included in a group depicting tuberculosis (irides 43-52). When these photographs were taken at the first consultation on 21.4.1940, the patient complained only of abdominal pain in the caecal region, stomach pressure and heartburn, as well as constipation and anal symptoms. On the second visit on 14.1.1941, he complained of chill and cough over the preceding three weeks, which had worsened during a visit to the Harz mountains, to which he had travelled for a change of air. Examination revealed pulmonary tuberculosis which was later confirmed by a chest specialist. The patient entered a sanatorium on 23.5.1941 and was not seen again. In March, 1951, the patient's mother reported that after some initial improvement, her son died after three years. The conduct of a life too unstable had caused his death.

What has the iris to say concerning this premature demise? Observing the right iris at 43-50', darker areas are seen with small catarrh signs (flakes at 43' and 47'—D). Similar small white catarrh signs are to be seen at 15', 16' and 17' in the pleural area, showing pulmonary encumbrance.

Still darker areas are shown at 23-28' and 31-33' corresponding to the position for the genital organs. Diametrically opposite, there

133

is a dark sector between 56′ and 3′ suggesting weakness of the cerebral functions and sexual over-activity. Assuming that the right iris especially reflects hereditary predisposition, then it can be taken in this case that a condition of sexual over-stimulation was transmitted. The small black points showing at 17′ and 19′ in the dorsal sector are not good signs.

The weakness of the respiratory organs is likewise shown in the left iris by the darkened areas at 10-17′ and 45-48′. The dark signs in the sector 23-33′ are especially noticeable. These signs, referring to the lower abdominal organs, not only refer to a disturbance of the descending colon and sigmoid flexure, but also show pathology affecting the left testicle.

The leg area at 30′ shows encumbrance, which considered together with the dark signs at 12-16′ in the heart area, suggests circulatory insufficiency. The long black sign at 37′ in the first major zone which appears to break through the iris-wreath, together with the fine black lines traversing the bladder area to the iris-rim and lying opposite to the white radials at 5-7′, needs no further explanation (refer to Iris-4) (E).

The large, dark areas in the upper quadrant of the iris between 55′ and 5′ in both irides show poor circulation to the brain. In all these irides showing a tubercular deterioration, it is to be appreciated that the tuberculosis is a consequence—not a cause.

Iris-53/54   **Male: right/left iris**

These irides show that a considerable degree of weakness affects all tissues, as may be seen in the loose-textured radial structure and the large lacunae.

The ring of white clouds around the iris-wreath in the third minor zone, are connected by thick white bands (lymph-bridges) to the ring of white flakes at the periphery. These white clouds and flakes are signs for inflammatory irritation of the lymphatic system and serous membrane encumbrance, so that repeated acute phases arise from chill, showing as colds, coughs and pleural irritation. Even the kidneys and peritoneum are involved.

Considering the first minor zone, it is seen that the stomach ring is also covered with white flakes (inflammation of the gastric mucosa). The white sign emphasis at the outer border of the stomach ring is found where stomach pains are strongly influenced by the weather (gastric rheumatism). The second minor zone likewise shows signs for mucous membrane catarrh. The peaked notches in this ring suggest that intestinal catarrh produces colicky pains and is the result of faulty nutrition.

Now to the signs in the right iris: Observing the first major zone, it is evident that the clouds and flakes are more intensely white in the sectors: 5-15', 25-35' and 40-50', suggesting that the inflammatory reaction is stronger in the parts projected in those areas. In sectors 5-15' and 40-50' the organs represented in the ciliary zone are concerned with respiration: 5-15'—nose, mouth, throat, neck and trachea, 40-50'—bronchi, lungs and pleura, and it is these organs which are repeatedly subject to pathological disturbances.

The particular indications at 18' are probably due to weakness of the back and pelvic tissues arising from an earlier injury (A). Were the organism free from poisonous toxins (metabolic residues) and were there to exist less over-relaxation of the skeletal structures, then inflammatory reactions in this region would be impossible. The same applies to the white clouds at 30' in the sector for feet.

The particularly intense white cloud at 35' indicates acute inflammation in the region for inguinal glands and peritoneum. How does this condition arise? To diagnose this correctly, observe the iris-wreath or the intestinal ring. At 35' the intestinal zone is widened and within this area is a small dark sign showing over-relaxation of the intestinal muscle layer with consequent local dilatation. Above and below the small, dark sign, small white flakes are to be seen, showing inflammation. The white radial lines running out from the intestine sign at first proceed in straight lines, but in traversing the third major zone they are seen to subdivide obliquely. These oblique lines indicate the presence of adhesions affecting this region (peritoneum). The intense white cloud is adjacent to an oblique line running to 30', showing that local inflammation, laxity and dilatation of the intestine, as well as adhesions of the intestine and peritoneum, are all involved (B).

At the first consultation the examination findings were as follows: omental rupture with inflammation and swelling of the inguinal glands. The omental rupture had been variously diagnosed as a cyst, an inguinal hernia, and as a cancerous nodule. The condition was in fact one of omental rupture which had been there for a long time. Since the caecum filled the hernial sack and the

135

appendix was involved, there was also a chronic inflammation of the appendix, hence the inguinal gland swelling.

At the time of the first consultation, the condition had already existed for six months. Since the patient had been investigated on several occasions and no operation had been advised, an attempt was made to relieve the inflammation by internal treatment and this was successful. A review of the condition after two months showed nothing more requiring attention and there were no other symptoms.

However, the signs in the second major zone between 20' and 28' probably show the true cause of the condition. In the fourth and fifth minor zones, prominent oblique white lines are found which indicate some earlier injury producing adhesions affecting the sacrum, coccyx and pelvic bones (C). Years before, the patient had fallen 15 metres and had broken both thigh and pelvic bones, which necessitated lying in plaster for six months.

It is thus not surprising if there had been lacerations within the abdominal cavity. The oblique lines at 35' are probably to be traced back to the injuries sustained at that time. If as the result of working activities the completely lax colon were subsequently to become involved with the scar-tissue, and inflammation of the appendix were to develop, then it would not give the typical syndrome of acute appendicitis, but pains would appear at intervals and swelling of the inguinal glands would be produced. Had the surgeon come to this conclusion, then he would certainly have decided to operate. Five years later, on my advice and after I had relieved the inflammation produced by the reappearing tumour, an operation was carried out.

Turning to the illustration of the left iris, transversals are also to be seen at 30-45' in the third major zone. Among these, a line goes from 42' at the iris-rim to 38' at the iris-wreath and then back again to the iris-rim at 34', thus forming a right angle directed towards the pupil (D). Transversals are likewise seen in the first major zone. Between 30' and 45' it also appears as though the stomach ring were compressed towards the pupillary margin.

The signs just described are all the result of injury. It is to be understood that both the back and the abdominal organs have been totally affected. The weakness and tissue laxity noted in the right iris is even more strongly shown in the left.

The signs for mouth and throat are also worse on the left than on the right. This fact implies that the patient has aggravated an already poor hereditary disposition by acquired conditions (mouth-hand line = nutrition line). The inherited tendency to disease of the respiratory organs is also strongly evident.

Iris-55/56   Male: 54 years—right/left iris

These irides are presented to corroborate the short explanation given for similar features appearing in Iris-28. Although the irides of the two patients do not completely agree, yet they have the same basic structure and organisation.

In more than 40 years of professional practice, only three patients have been seen with irides showing these particular features. Patient-28 is still alive. On my advice, he modified his way of life and undertook a course of basic treatment. The second patient attended only once and no further information is available.

The patient now being considered attended for his first consultation on 11.3.1939. As the case record indicates, he complained of severe burning pains in the stomach which referred up into the throat, total constipation, attacks of cardiac cramp and pains over the whole body. According to his statement, the attending physician had been treating him for stomach neuralgia and cardiac neurosis. A radiograph taken shortly before he came was apparently negative for ulcer or cancer. The general body pains had been treated for years as rheumatism.

The irisdiagnosis findings were: general infection, gastric ulceration with involvement of the pancreas, and coronary sclerosis. After five treatment sessions, during which time there was some initial improvement in the stomach symptoms, the patient was referred for in-patient treatment. His wife later reported that he was sent into hospital by his panel doctor in September 1939. The first operation on the 9th September confirmed cancer of the stomach. After some initial improvement, the patient was again submitted for surgical treatment during 1940, which revealed that extensive metastases affected all abdominal organs. In the last few days before he died, there was total decompensation, urine and faeces were just pus and stinking excreta and there was purulent disintegration of the skin and subcutaneous tissues.

The patient was 54 years old in 1939, the fifth child of nine

137

siblings. He was a post-office clerk, married with two children. The father died at the age of 49 years from joint rheumatism and the mother at 59 years of age from cardiac weakness.

Part 2

MEDICATION AND PROGNOSIS

A. W. Priest

FOREWORD

Irisdiagnosis is not a matter of arriving at some medical 'name' and then proceeding to consider the herbal and biochemic medicines commonly used empirically for such named conditions. Naturopathic medication is a direct correlation of the properties of natural medicines with the disturbances shown in the iris. It thus constitutes treatment which is entirely individual to the patient. Indeed, the 'label' is both superfluous and irrelevant.

In Part 2 of the text, there is no attempt to be exhaustive or to discuss the detailed treatment of the individual cases presented in Part 1. The object of this section is to elucidate those basic principles of medication which can be applied and adapted to individual needs, using the herbal and biochemic medicines in common professional use.

The remedies suggested are representative of the qualities required, not specific for diseases, and there are many possible alternatives to those named. Herbal medicines are generally referred to by the genus name only, the species being assumed to be that usually prescribed. Precise details of these agents are given in—*'Herbal Medication—a Clinical and Dispensary Handbook'*— A. W. and L. R. Priest, London, 1982, L. N. Fowler and Co. Ltd., to which the reader may refer as a companion volume for information concerning the materia medica.

The unique value of irisdiagnosis is to provide a therapeutic perspective and indicate the individual prognosis.

London, 1984.   A. W. Priest.

Contents

BASIC SIGNS AND VALUES

The symptoms presented by a patient are not a complete indicator of the basic organismic condition. The larger part of disease change proceeds insidiously and only when such processes exhaust the capacity of the organism to accommodate these changes and encroach acutely upon some vital process do symptoms appear. Symptoms are merely the point of stress and may be relatively remote from the true centre of disease. The functional output of the kidney or the vital capacity of the lungs can be considerably reduced before symptoms appear.

The difficulty in any clinical investigation of the patient's condition is to arrive at a true perspective of the total state of health, to relate the findings of interrogation and examination in such a way as to provide a clear picture of the pathological processes at work. Failing achievement of this perspective, treatment inevitably deteriorates into the mere relief or suppression of symptoms and the recourse to empiricism.

The value of irisdiagnosis in this context is in the correlation of tissue and functional conditions, in providing that basic assessment necessary before the treatment of conditions, rather than symptoms, can proceed. It is not the purpose of irisdiagnosis to do those things which can be more exactly measured by physical and laboratory procedures, but to provide the overall perspective for clinical control and therapeutic direction.

Physiological basis

The aim of a more advanced study of irisdiagnosis is to acquire this deeper perspective, to develop that synthetic approach to iris-analysis to which Theodor Kriege refers in his own introduction. Diagnosis in this sense has little to do with an allopathic appellation—the 'name' of the disease. Since irisdiagnosis is largely a method of 'horizontal'* assessment, then it reveals the evolution of the pathological state in the patient being considered. The very fact of an iris-sign means that the causative conditions for its appearance have existed for some time and the more chronic the sign indication, the longer have those conditions existed. Indeed, once there are structural signs present in the iris, they will persist

*Priest, A. W. and Priest, L. R. (1982) *Herbal Medication,* L. N. Fowler & Co. Ltd. London.

147

for the remainder of life, although the functional conditions to which they pertain may have been resolved.

By the same token, fleeting changes and transitory conditions of relatively short duration will not register in the iris. Since iris-signs arise largely on the basis of autonomic nervous reflexes, then the tissue integrity of the iris-fibres will be resistant to transitory reflex influences. Only the constant and continuous impulse will register.

At a more primitive level of animal function the organism relies upon humoral mechanisms, upon the interaction of chemical substances in solution. But this essentially intra-cellular mechanism is less immediately adaptable to organismic function in the more complex multi-cellular systems of man, so that even with the elaboration of humoral control by endocrine functions, the ultimate means of co-ordination consist of the neuro-endocrine system and the autonomic motor/vasomotor functions. It is on the basis of these two organismic control systems that iris-signs arise, thus:

(1) Humoral signs: colour changes and pigment depositions which are topolabile.

(2) Reflex signs: functional and structural changes affecting the iris-fibres, both radial and circular, which are topostabile.

Therapeutic objectives

Accordingly, treatment needs to be both humoral and physiological. Humoral regulation is concerned with the qualitative aspects of the blood and body fluids, with problems of systemic encumbrance from autotoxaemia and the vital state generally, whereas the objectives in physiological treatment are to restore functional equilibrium and optimum trophic state to the bodily organs and systems.

Proper nutrition and alimentation, in which the end products of protein and carbohydrate metabolism are minimised, is the foundation of naturopathic treatment, and such an approach will be adequate where digestive and eliminative organs are normal. However, failing a normal functional capacity of these organs, the recovery of health will be but partial and some degree of disability will remain.

It is in the assessment of physiological limitations that irisdiagnosis is so valuable, in providing visual evidence of

148

functional disturbance and organic weakness affecting specific organs and systems, so that with suitable medication over-contracted conditions may be relaxed, over-relaxed conditions toned, and the functional capacity and structural integrity of organs and tissues restored to the optimum possible.

It is evident from these considerations that there is a natural order of treatment to be reviewed under the following headings—

(1) Nutrition and the state of the digestive functions.
(2) The adequacy of the eliminative functions and the state of encumbrance.
(3) The equilibrium of the nervous and circulatory systems to ensure proper control and distribution of circulating fluids.
(4) The functional and structural capacity of specific organs.

Sign evaluation

The great advantage of irisdiagnosis over other systems of reflex analysis is in its accessibility. Indeed, the broad indications may be noted under normal lighting conditions and unknown to the patient. However, some degree of magnification and focal illumination is necessary for clinical examination, although the microscopical detail obtainable with a corneal microscope is unnecessary for ordinary assessment. Magnifications of ×4 to ×10 are adequate, remembering that contrast values diminish as magnification increases.

Although there is continuous research to establish the physiological connections between the iris and the body systems, the interpretation can be considered holistically in terms of symbolic values, thus—

(1) As a circle, the iris expresses balance. Disturbances of functional equilibrium are shown by departures from the circular form. Physiological response in the organism is the function of the nervous system, hence disturbances reflect in aberrations of contraction/relaxation which affect the circular representations in the iris.
(pupil, iris-wreath, nerve rings, radii solaris, iris-margin)
(2) The iris fibres and layers represent disturbances of structure and relationship. Since structure affects function and reflects integrity, then texture has come to represent organic resistance.

(lacunae, crypts, honeycomb signs, defect signs, textural looseness)

(3) The distribution of light and shade indicates vital reactivity, in which light symbolises life and dark represents decline. Thus, white signs show active response of a constructive, resistant or resolvent quality, while black signs indicate tissue degeneration or destruction.
(white flakes, wisps, clouds, radials, sign-borders).

Thus, the simple indicators are:

Circle	=	Function	—	Equilibrium/imbalance
Texture	=	Structure	—	Integrity/resistance
Light/shade	=	Reactivity	—	Vitality/encumbrance.

Signs of circular or segmental representation are directly indicative of nervous imbalance, involving either the central or autonomic nervous systems. Thus, ovular distortion of the pupil reflects central nervous disturbance, whereas sectoral flattening of the pupillary margin suggests localised involvement of spinal segmental reflexes (sympathetic outflow). The distortions of the iris-wreath directly reflect sympathetic/parasympathetic imbalance as affecting the part of the gut or organ represented in the sector concerned. Likewise, nerve rings are typical of an anxiety background and radii solaris may suggest spasmophilia.

Texture represents trophicity, especially of connective tissue. Since connective tissue is the structural basis for all organs and vital tissues, then to this extent functional sufficiency depends upon structural integrity. The narrow context in which structural relationships are commonly considered, that is, in terms of the gross structures, completely overlooks the part played by the trabecular skeleton of all vital organs. Generally and locally, iris textural indications show the state of the connective tissues, especially the first and immediately visible stromal layer. The integrity of this layer indicates those inherited and acquired factors of insufficiency and weakness in the metabolism of the substances necessary in structural tissues, especially the calcium salts and the silicates.

Just as the outer stromal layer of the iris represents the connective tissue structures, so the deeper stromal layer, the vascular, is taken to indicate the integrity of the parenchymatous cells. Since the vascular stromal layer is thick, individual structural signs can show an increasing depth down to the retinal layer, which ultimately appears as dark-brown or dark-grey to black in colour. The completely degenerated condition of this ultimate degree of penetration represents necrosis or mummification and suggests that tissue recovery in the affected organ is no longer possible.

It is important in the case of all structural signs to note whether associated signs (white) indicate acute activity, either in the organ itself or involving contiguous structures. Likewise, local depositions of colour pigment may suggest degenerative or malignant change, and the presence of transversals indicate adhesions or displacements.

However, the shape or extent of any sign has no absolute value, but must be assessed against the context of the general background. As Theodor Kriege states in relation to heart signs (lacunae—Iris 32A), a large sign does not necessarily indicate dilatation. In the fine textured iris, the smallest deviation of structure should be regarded as significant.

Similarly, there is no fixed and absolute position for any organ location, even though the typical signs are considered topostabile. Ciliary zone signs are subject to displacement from distortions of the iris-wreath (Iris 7F), the effects of visceral displacement (Iris 16D, 19J, 6CD), or the widthwise extension of a large sign (possible tumour formation—Iris 43F, 45F), and in any case all sign areas overlap. The topography of the uterus, kidneys and other abdominal organs is variable within fairly wide limits, so that final judgment may rest upon the existence of other signs and indications. Finally, the surface structures may be so completely distorted as to render detailed interpretation unreliable ('ox-eye daisy' iris).

Structural signs

There is some apparent confusion in relation to the common structural signs, since the literature may refer to all as 'defect-signs' or 'loss-of-substance signs'. These signs are properly referred to as—lacunae, crypts, honeycomb signs and defect signs—and each may be properly defined.

Lacunae: Lacunae, otherwise known as weakness-signs, are signs of variable width and extension. Typically, the limits of the sign are represented by arc-lines originating at an inner point and curving outwards towards the periphery. If the arc-lines meet to form a closed, oval shape, the lacuna is described as 'closed'. (Iris 16) In an 'open' lacuna, the arc-lines remain apart and may deviate in any direction or diffuse into the general stroma (Iris 39).

The lacuna always indicates weakness and hypofunction. In its simplest form, it affects only the surface layer, the connective tissue layer, and suggests an early degree of trophic insufficiency without pathological erosion of the parenchymatous elements. The closed lacuna indicates a fully compensated condition in which there is no longer any active disease process or progressive degeneration, especially when the sign is surrounded by a definite but thin white border (healed lesion—Iris 16F). A much thicker border which encloses only part of the sign, or diffuses into the surrounding area as a white cloud, suggests inflammatory irritation of the contiguous structures and is a more common feature of the open lacuna (Iris 45F). Direct treatment for the organ represented by a closed lacuna is not indicated, although the reduced functional reserve has to be allowed for as an organ-inferiority.

The open lacuna is to be regarded as an indication of progressive trophic deterioration which may be influenced by constructive treatment and trophorestorative medication. However, the functional incapacity is to be considered latent and may not become evident as a clinical symptom until environmental stresses make excessive demands upon the reduced reserve. Thus, clinical evidence may not be apparent until organ damage, infection or aging has occurred, although sudden organ failure is always a possibility.

In the typical oval shape of a lacuna, the greatest width is less than the overall length of the sign. Increased width, especially when greater than the length, indicates stasis, swelling or tumour formation of the organ or part concerned (Iris 46GH).

Crypts: Crypts are square- or rhomboid-shaped 'holes' affecting the deeper stromal layer. Just as the ovular shape of the typical lacuna arises from the radial fibres of the surface layer, so the shape of the crypt is due to the criss-cross interlacing network of the vascular stroma. Thus, crypts indicate involvement of the essential functional cells of an organ, the parenchymatous and glandular elements which subserve its particular function.

The upper stromal layer extends from the iris-wreath to the outer rim. The iris fibres visible in the first major zone, the gastro-intestinal, are those of the deeper stromal layer, so that the typical structural signs appearing in this zone are crypts and defect-signs, indicating essential cell damage. Functional conditions of over-contraction and over-relaxation affecting the gut are shown rather by the state of the iris-wreath (the inner edge of the connective-tissue stroma) than by changes affecting the vascular stroma and so visible within the zone. Crypts usually indicate ulcerative or necrotic processes with a tendency to perforation when appearing in the gastro-intestinal zone. (Iris 16D)

Honeycomb signs: These signs might be regarded as midway between lacunae and crypts. The sign consists of a group of small square-shaped cavities which may occasionally appear as an individual sign, but is more likely to be seen as honeycomb-like formations within a lacuna, thus showing deterioration from the simple lacuna formation in which the radial fibres are still visible.

Honeycomb signs are considered to be indications of simple atrophy or cirrhosis secondary to vaso-motor disturbance. Interpretation will be coloured by the location in which they are found. Thus, in the intestinal zone adhesions are likely, whereas in skeletal areas osteoporosis is a possible condition (Iris 32B, 36G). An organ inferiority with functional insufficiency is always indicated.

Defect signs: Defect signs are small points, lines or fissures observed between the radial fibres. They will appear dark or black according to the degree of penetration down to the basal layer. Although such signs may appear singly as part of a textural loosening, they more often appear within lacunae, crypts or honeycomb signs to show the presence of focal degenerative processes.

Principles of Medication

Iris diagnosis thus provides the basis for appropriate treatment. While the usual clinical methods can reveal the extent of functional disturbance at the time of examination ('vertical' assessment), they cannot directly indicate the background capacity of the organ systems, nor the constitutional tendencies or vital response

153

('horizontal' assessment), and these important considerations must otherwise be assessed by deduction from the case history—a faculty requiring considerable clinical maturity.

Whatever the presenting syndrome, every medicinal prescription must take into account the following factors—

(1) the constitutional texture and response,
(2) the reserve capacity of the vital organs, and
(3) the amount or degree of toxic encumbrance and systemic obstruction.

Since textural integrity represents general vitality and resistance and is an index of response and recuperative power, then observation of iris texture decides the orientation of medicinal treatment, thus—

(1) the worse the texture, the longer must be the restorative programme and the greater emphasis placed upon long-term trophic recovery;
(2) the worse the texture, the more that strongly alterative agents are to be used with caution and the slower any promotion of toxic elimination.

All vital organs possess considerable functional reserve, which is drawn upon to meet excessive or prolonged demand. A reduction in this reserve capacity arising from trophic insufficiency or some insidious pathological process may not be clinically evident and yet must be considered when stimulating the affected organ to increased function for the purpose of relieving or resolving some systemic condition. Thus, the strong stimulation of increased heart, liver or kidney function to resolve rheumatic syndromes could produce organ embarrassment if reserve capacity is lacking. The stimulus value of the prescription must be well within the organ capacity.

Toxic encumbrance, giving rise to systemic obstruction, consists of the precipitation of waste products and unusable chemical compounds into intercellular spaces. The reduction of vital response resulting from sedative and depressant drugs, whether from habitual use or by way of suppressive treatment of acute eliminative phases, means that the essential disease process extends further before the onset of active resistance and the mobilisation of

154

eliminative resources. In showing the degree of encumbrance, irisdiagnosis enables the practitioner to assess whether the positive promotion of an eliminative crisis by powerful herbal alteratives should be deferred or avoided.

In general, medicinal treatment for chronic conditions should observe the following order of priority considerations:

(1) Support organ inferiorities, especially vital organs.
(2) Promote gentle systemic trophorestoration.
(3) Adopt a controlled programme of toxic resolution, especially of old foci of suppressed infections.

The medicinal substances used in the naturopathic treatment of functional and organic disorders consist of mineral and plant materials. The mineral elements forming part of the body's own structure, together with those which are basic to the formation and interaction of natural chemical compounds within the organism, are prepared in such a way (homoeopathic potentisation) as to facilitate absorption and activation. The carbonates, chlorides, phosphates and sulphates of the metals: calcium, magnesium, potassium and sodium (extended Schuessler biochemic series), together with the salts of iron, copper, silica and other trace elements, provide the basis for humoral regulation and the restoration of systemic and tissue deficiencies.

Plant medicines are used as nutritional, humoral and physiological remedies. It should be decided at the outset whether the intention is to—

(1) supply material quantities to supplement nutritional sources,
(2) regulate systemic balance and function through the physiological systems, or
(3) restore the tissue integrity and trophic capacity of some particular organ, so far as may be possible,

—since the intention will determine the dosage level in terms of potency, quantity and duration. Relatively large quantities of infusions and decoctions are necessary for supplying mineral salts and other nutritional properties, whereas tinctures and fluid extracts are the usual medium for influencing function and regulating the systems. The long-term, low-level dosage needed for the gradual improvement of organ integrity and capacity is best administered in the form of drops, pills or tablets. In this respect, the use of low potency preparations ($1\times$ to $3\times$) of fresh plant materials may be preferred.

ALIMENTARY PROCESSES

Iris-signs representing the gastro-intestinal tract reflect the symbolic interpretations particularly well:

(1) Departures from the circular form to indicate disturbances of functional equilibrium affecting the autonomic nervous system.
(2) Textural and structural changes from disturbed vaso-motor reflexes showing the trophic state of the viscera.
(3) Variations of colour, white to black, to indicate the degree of vital reactivity, together with pigment deposits to reveal disturbed enzyme function.

Circular form

The pupil normally contracts and dilates freely, so that undue and persistent contraction or dilatation will indicate disturbance of the central or autonomic nervous system. Dilatation of the pupil results from sympathetic nerve impulses, whereas contraction of the pupil is due to parasympathetic impulses. A protracted condition of miosis (pupillary contraction) arises from an irritated state of the parasympathetic or a paralytic state of the sympathetic system. Pupillary contraction is a common feature of old age (senile miosis) and is also to be found when certain drugs are being used. Where there are no such influences to be taken into account, the contracted pupil may indicate a general tendency to spasmophilic conditions, including spasm of the intestinal tract, globus hystericus, tetany, etc. (Iris 22, 29).

Widely dilated pupils are signs of increased sympathetic tonus. Associated with wide eyelids and protruding eyeballs, the dilatation is characteristic of hyperthyroid conditions. Physiological stimulation of the sympathetic system, as in the invasive stage of fevers, will also produce dilatation. A temporary aggravation of the dilatation typically seen in young children must be allowed for in interpretation and in attempting to photograph the young iris. It is a good plan to fire the flash gun once or twice before taking the actual photograph, to induce the pupil to contract. In any case, a preliminary inspection in good natural light should be made before exhibiting apparatus which would be likely to produce anxiety.

There is no question that the most common presenter of the

dilated pupil is the patient of asthenic type. The association with chronic sympatheticotonia is obvious, and indicates that the organism is under stress from chronic nutritional insufficiency. There could be no better example of a vicious circle, since the existence of the sympathetic emphasis is the very factor which inhibits expansion of digestion and absorption. To produce a positive weight increase in such conditions is a most difficult clinical achievement. The deeply entrenched anxiety pattern so often found is both a cause and an effect of the asthenic condition.

The iris-wreath is normally without irregularity of colour, shape or plasticity, encircling the wreath zone with an even rhythm of undulation. Deviations of the circular form inwards or outwards show functional disturbance of the gastro-intestinal system. A totally contracted or expanded wreath zone is shown when the iris-wreath is positioned nearer or farther from the pupil (Iris 11 and 12 compare). Local variations in the width of the wreath zone are traditionally correlated with the tone of the gut, in which narrowing represents contraction and widening signifies laxity. The trophic state of the tissues is indicated by the integrity of the iris fibres in the wreath zone (gastro-intestinal zone) and of the wreath itself.

The contracted iris-wreath suggests irritability and hypertonicity. A total narrowing of the wreath zone with small pupil and forward bulging of the iris is characteristic of the spasmophilia seen in the hypersthenic habitus type. Narrowing of the wreath zone in the frontal quadrant of the iris suggests ptosis of the transverse colon (Iris 9, 27). Sharply contracted sections of the wreath indicate local visceral constriction, possibly arising from adhesions or injury (Iris 18A, 19AG), especially when the sign appears as a wedge pointing towards the pupil. It is possible for the iris-wreath to be so contracted as completely to cover the first major zone (Iris 2, 29, 55-56) and frequently to obscure the second minor zone (intestinal ring).

The dilated wreath-zone indicates relative weakness, atonicity of the gut, and is often very marked in the areas for caecum, hepatic flexure and descending colon (Iris 7—descending colon, Iris 10—hepatic flexure, Iris 12—caecum). Marked dilatation of the wreath opposite the heart area in the left iris signifies Roemheld syndrome (atonic constipation with gas formation and pressure on contiguous structures, especially the heart (Iris 5, 9, 26D). Partial dilatation is usually accompanied by textural weakness (fibre looseness) in the same sector, showing that the condition is hypotrophic as well as atonic.

Structural lesions and textural signs

Increased or reduced tonicity (over-contracted or over-relaxed) must in due course affect the trophic state. Tissue nutrition depends upon a proper balance of function and either extreme of disturbance will gradually produce degenerative changes. The integrity of systemic and organ tissues will be reflected in the iris areas, together with indications of vital response (light and shade).

In the presence of specific symptoms, the search for focal organ lesions must not overlook the general textural changes in the areas concerned. Symptoms arise when functional capacity reduces below the minimum level required from an organ, yet there may be no evidence of a focal lesion to account for the symptoms. Similarly, dark colouring may indicate sub-function from sclerotic degeneration, even though no structural signs or textural changes are evident.

Textural changes affecting the iris-fibres in the gastro-intestinal zone involve the second (deeper) stromal layer. When organ signs in the ciliary zones, the second and third major zones, penetrate to the second layer, it is taken to mean that there is some degree of essential tissue damage (crypts, defect-signs) as distinct from the tendency to functional weakness or reduced capacity indicated when the sign penetrates no further than the first layer (lacunae). Thus, all tissue signs in the wreath zone are to be read as organic signs. In this zone, fibre loosening, defect signs and crypts represent loss of organic integrity affecting secretory glands and motor elements.

Correspondingly, lesioned organs may be symptomless if functional capacity is adequate and the organ capsule unaffected by the local disturbance. Purely parenchymatous lesions are often symptomless, hence destructive changes in the duodenum, liver or pancreas may be indicated by iris-signs in the absence of subjective symptoms.

Defect signs, also known as loss-of-substance signs, are easily visible at relatively low magnifications and appear as points, streaks and tears of variable width which penetrate deeply into the stromal layer. The chronicity of a focal ulcer may be determined by

159

assessing the depth of erosion into the tissue. These signs follow the radial course of the iris-fibres (Iris 8, 17, 23, 24, 45).

The more serious defects are shown by very deep signs which are wedge-, torpedo- or rhomboid-shaped. Wedge-signs are typical of ulcer formation, in which case there may be a white colouring of the stomach ring to indicate hyperchlorhydria (Iris 12A, 20A). Malignant changes are more likely with rhomboid and torpedo signs when the stomach ring is basically dark in colour, although superimposed islands of white may suggest secondary fermentative dyspepsia (lactic acid formation). (Iris 17, 21, 23, 24).

Light and shade

The colour of the wreath-zone may vary from a brilliant white to almost black. The natural colour is considered to be light grey for the circular stomach ring (first minor zone) to indicate normal acidity of the gastric secretion. The development of partial or total lightening of colour indicates an increased tendency to hyper-acidity as the colour lifts towards a brilliant white (Iris 11, 12).

The colour of defect-signs will vary from dark grey to black, representing tissue destruction, and this colour will persist even after healing (ulcers, etc.). The colour of a declining gastric function is not so dark as that of defect-signs, varying from grey to dark-grey as the acidity level falls off from normal to hypo-acidity and anacidity. It will be recalled that pepsin is only active in the presence of hydrochloric acid, and that calcium absorption also depends upon adequate acidity. Thus, the assessment of the gastric capacity from the basic colour of the stomach ring is important in all problems of under-nutrition and in the asthenic constitution generally.

The variation of colour from white to black is accompanied by a change of tissue level, being raised in acute conditions (white signs) and sunken in chronic destructive conditions. (Good vision of these fine differences requires rather high magnification with stereoscopic facility.) In the presence of structural signs the basic colour of the zone has differential value. Where there is intense white colouring and a contracted wreath it is probable that the signs refer to ulcers, whereas a generally dark background increases the chance of malignant change. Ulcer erosion is more likely in the presence of hyperchlorhydria, whereas malignant change favours anacid conditions.

160

The stomach ring

The stomach ring is more or less easily identified, the ring area corresponding directly with the position of the M. sphincter pupillae. Close examination of the stomach ring in the illustrations shows that its position and uniformity is maintained in spite of the highly variable position of the iris-wreath, even where it has been overlapped by the wreath line (Iris 12, 43-44).

Theoretically, the first major zone is equally divided to form the stomach and intestinal zones, so that the width of the intestinal is roughly equal to that of the stomach zone. In many of the illustrations this is far from being the case, the width of the intestinal zone varying greatly according to the wreath position, totally or segmentally. Where the wreath contracts inwards as far as the outer edge of the stomach ring, then the intestinal zone is completely obscured, in which case signs immediately adjacent to the outer margin of the wreath and overlying the normal position for the intestinal zone may be interpreted as intestinal signs rather than metabolic (minor zone 3), especially where the outer iris layer is obviously thin and attenuated (Iris 43-44). It will help to differentiate these indications if it is remembered that stomach and intestine signs are second layer signs. Only the first stromal layer is so highly variable.

Interpretation and medication

Irisdiagnosis is not a matter of arriving at some medical 'name' and then proceding to consider the herbal medicines commonly used empirically for such named conditions. Correct treatment is a direct correlation of the vital, humoral and physiological properties of natural medicines with those disturbances shown in the iris. It thus constitutes treatment which is individual to the patient. Indeed, the 'label' is both superfluous and irrelevant.

The iris-signs themselves suggest the remedial influences needed—

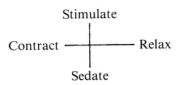

Over active conditions will require sedating or diffusing, while subactive responses need stimulating. Over-contracted states of viscero-motor or vaso-motor function require relaxing, whereas over-relaxed conditions need toning. These functional corrections can be achieved with appropriate medication on a more or less short-term basis.

Rather longer time is needed for the treatment of conditions evidenced by structural signs. The decline of essential tissue integrity suggested by all defect-signs dictates a careful programme of trophorestorative influence and a respect for the existing reduced organ capacity. The depth and extent of the sign becomes a measure of prognosis.

A direct and immediate correlation is available to meet the typical conditions encountered in clinical practice, assuming that the symptoms accord with the iris indications—

(1) Tissue tonics and trophorestoratives in over-relaxed conditions such as gastroptosis, visceroptosis, etc. Agents such as Calc.fluor., Calc.phos., Silicea in low potency, and the herbal medicines: Juglans cinerea, Uva-ursi, Myrica, etc., are appropriate for the connective tissue weakness.

(2) Soothing demulcents for irritable and inflamed mucosal conditions, shown by increased whiteness close around the pupil—Altheae rad., Symphytum rad., Ulmus fulva, etc.

(3) Stimulant tonics for deficient gastric secretory functions— Alpinia, Rosmarinus, Xanthoxylum, and the bitter tonics—indicated by increased darkness of the stomach ring.

(4) Autonomic relaxants for hypermotility and over-contraction of the digestive apparatus secondary to a general parasympatheticotonia, suggested by an over-contracted iris-wreath and a small pupil—Dioscorea, Matricaria, etc.

(5) Trophorestorative tonics with gentle stimulants for hypomotility and over-relaxation of the intestines suggested by an outward dilatation of the iris-wreath—Juglans cin., Hydrastis, Xanthoxylum, Calc.carb., Calc.fluor., etc.

This ready clinical approach enables treatment to be commenced at a relatively superficial level while detailed investigations are pursued and a more profound study of the individual patient is being made. It will be appreciated that iris-sign interpretation is not a matter of spot-diagnosis. The deeper perspective advocated by Theodor Kriege, as portrayed in his own interpretations, requires time for thought and review, in order to achieve a balanced schema of medication.

Typical syndromes

The association of certain symptoms and conditions into typical syndromes provides a basis for differential evaluation and medication—

(1) The acute gastric condition with hyperchlorhydria and the onset of diffuse or focal ulceration with maximal symptoms.
(2) Chronic pyloric-duodenal ulceration with adhesions and obstruction, often with minimal symptoms.
(3) Digestive insufficiency and poor assimilation from spastic, atrophic and indurated states of the intestine with or without secondary toxic absorption.
(4) Degenerative changes with potential malignancy.

Acute stomach: The acute state with hyperchlorhydria is well shown in iris illustrations 11, 12, 22 and 27, in which there is also the contracted wreath or small pupil typical of parasympathetic emphasis. Whether expressing a general hypersthenic background or reflecting a specific psychosomatic stress, it is the vagotonia which is the immediate objective in treatment. The over-contracted and irritable stomach needs the strong relaxation provided by say Dioscorea, reinforced as necessary by Cypripedium or even Lobelia. Acute but short exacerbations may be helped with Mag.phos.

The hyperchlorhydria as such calls for Spiraea as the best influence to regulate gastric acidity. Since potential or actual ulceration is present, the remedy is best given as an infusion, in order to avoid aggravation by the alcohol content of herbal tinctures or fluid extracts. Actual ulceration in the acute stage needs the demulcent influence of Ulmus fulva or Symphytum, given as a gruel. A very small quantity of powdered extracts of Hydrastis and Calendula added to the Ulmus fulva will supplement the healing influence. A restrictive or mono-diet is necessary.

Treatment of the acute phase must gradually change to meet the deeper causes and conditions as the acute symptoms are relieved. Iris-11 suggests that the autonomic stress arises from an endocrine disturbance (pituitary and suprarenal signs) rather than a typological emphasis, and a psychosomatic or endocrine

163

investigation is needed for individualising treatment. Similarly for Iris 27.

In Iris-12, vagal irritability is shown by the thick white segments of the iris-wreath, rather than by a total contraction, in view of the very poor textural (trophic) state. The white wedge signs (12A) are not deep and suggest a relatively recent development for the ulcerated condition of the stomach. Nevertheless, the poor textural background indicates a much slower response to medication, and connective tissue tonics are needed—Symphytum rad., rather than Ulmus fulva for the gruel, Calc.carb., Calc.phos., etc., as well as Ferr.phos. for susceptibility to chill.

Iris 22 shows greater deterioration and more profound nervous disturbance with potential malignancy. Medication can do no more than to relieve the symptoms.

Associated problems may emerge to dominate treatment. The existence of adhesions (transversals) may severely limit response. External pressure (Iris-15) or old injury (Iris-18) may complicate. Rheumatic influences producing stomach cramp, shown by strong white demarcation of the outer border of the stomach ring, suggest the inclusion of Ballota nig. or even more powerful antispasmodics in the prescription, together with Xanthoxylum if the stomach can tolerate the stimulus.

Chronic duodenum: Chronic ulceration of pylorus and duodenum may show minimal symptoms. An insidiously developing digestive insufficiency with sporadic sub-acute phases can accompany a considerable pyloric-duodenal erosion. Indeed, unexpected haemorrhage may be the first intimation (Iris 17).

The typological background is often quite different to that commonly associated with hyperchlorhydria, and may indeed suggest asthenic sympatheticotonia with an anxiety basis (Iris-9/10—large pupil, nerve rings and suprarenal signs, aggravated by spinal-coccygeal injury). Such a background induces over-contraction of the gastro-intestinal sphincters, especially pylorus-duodenum, and indicates the need for Pulsatilla as part of the prescription.

Undoubtedly, the most complicating feature of chronic duodenal ulceration is the development of adhesions to contiguous organs and structures, especially those implicating the pancreas (13C, 18C, 19D), or liver-gallbladder (17B, 25A, 41R), involving back-pressure upon the biliary and pancreatic secretions. If the adhesions consist of no more than inflammatory agglutinations, suggested by lightly marked transversals or cobweb signs, then careful visceral manipulative techniques or long-fasting may be successful in the hands of those especially skilled in such procedures. Otherwise, fibrous adhesions may require surgical treatment when obstruction occurs. The onset of eczematous conditions, or other metabolic indications of disturbed liver function, should sound a warning. Meanwhile, beyond treatment for the acute exacerbations, medicines should maintain sphincter relaxation (Chelidonium, Dioscorea, Kali phos) and clear catarrhal congestion (Chionanthes, Berberis vulg./aquif., Hydrastis, Kali mur., Kali sulph.).

Alimentary insufficiency: Digestive insufficiency with poor assimilation inevitably arises from chronic inflammatory and ulcerative conditions following the development of scar tissue and cicatrisation. The increased darkness and depth of the signs and lesions in the gastro-intestinal zone of the iris indicates the transition from hyperfunction to debility and insufficiency. The coarse striations show the mucosal decline and the development of adhesions inhibits peristalsis or gives rise to obstructive colic.

Conditions of chronic gastric sub-acidity, hypochlorhydria, may be read from the following iris indications, especially if there is a general complaint of a sense of fullness after meals containing much protein:

(1) a dark-grey gastro-intestinal zone,
(2) brown pigmentation in a blue or grey iris (central heterochromia),
(3) defect-signs in the first major zone—black points, streaks or tears.

Iris-14 is typical of such a condition of hypoacidity from organic degeneration. Illustrations 45 and 47 show a more severe degree of deterioration of the gastric mucosa in the radiating black/white lines suggesting a coarsened structure.

Spasticity of the gastro-intestinal tract, even where there is a dilated pupil, must result in atrophic changes from prolonged vaso-constriction and ultimate chronic innutrition and induration (Iris 9D, 5B, 10F). In spite of the potential onset of malignant degeneration evident in illustrations 21, 22 and 23, the nutritional

165

insufficiency must be kept in mind. There is here a case for supplementation with dilute hydrochloric acid, pepsin, papain, and pancreatin, and dietetic adjustment to provide easily absorbed foods to minimise digestive demands. Mild trophorestorative medication: Alpinia, Berberis aquif., Chionanthes, Hydrastis and Verbena, together with moderately relaxing influences are indicated.

The most serious complication is the toxic absorption of the products of incomplete digestive processing through the damaged mucosal layer, with the consequent development of peripheral saturation (encumbrance), lymphatic obstruction and allergic responses. In this respect note Theodor Kriege's own comparison of Iris-28 and Iris-29. Dietetic adjustment to minimise fermentation and putrefaction of the content of the gut by feeding proteins and starches at separate meals and avoiding combinations of starches with acid fruits at the same meal (Hay diet principles—after Dr. W. H. Hay) will do much to assist. Meanwhile, antiseptic medication and agents to assist lymphatic function are indicated: Baptisia, Echinacea, Myrrha, Phytolacca. etc.

Degenerative changes: Degenerative conditions and latent or actual malignancy will be suggested by deep substance signs: rhomboid-signs, torpedo-signs and deep wedge-signs. Illustration 14 shows dark wedge-signs and deeply scored black lines suggestive of malignant development. (Iris 17, 22, 23, 40.) Illustrations 55-56 indicate impending dissolution from total metastatic malignant degeneration.

Neurasthenic ring: light brown ring directly around the pupil (uveal seam).

Neurogenous: name for blue iris.

Open weakness marks: similar to lacunae in occurrence and appearance — mostly not chambered, open or closed at the edge, distinguished from lacunae by the upper layer which is only darkened and not displaced or destroyed.

Parchment rolls: see congestion furrows.

Radials: blood vessels which appear as spoke-like cords in the iris and run from the frill up to the edge of the iris.

String frill: see frill, in this case looking like an expanded string.

Solar rays: very thin, dark, line-type structures, mostly in the blue and mixed iris, running outwards from the pupil, mostly cranial — and can run parallel with the radials right up to the edge of the iris.

Transversals: sideways running radials — light — pigmented — vascularised (red)

Tophi: white close flecks in the blue and mixed iris. Smooth but also irregular edging possible, often pigmented.

Wisps: similar to tophi, but more transparent.

Central Heterochromia: obviously darker, pigmented central part of the iris around the pupil and frill; stands out well from the peripheral lighter part of the iris.

Central Pigmentation: see central heterochromia.

Ciliary Area: name for the part of the iris between the frill and the edge of the iris.

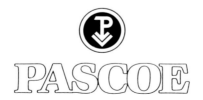

GLOSSARY OF TERMS

Blood and Lymph region: approx. a 1 mm wide circular zone directly around the frill.

Dyscrasia: toxic blood and lymphatic disorder.

Skin Ring: dark edge to iris, can be between 1 to 3 mm wide.

Haematogenic: name for the dark brown iris, without stroma markings.

Hydrogenic Constitution: tendency to illness in cold, damp weather.

Iris stroma: structural name for the part of the iris between the frill and the edge of the iris.

Cramp Rings: circular, light fold formations, also called circular contraction furrows — in all variations on the circular — semi- and quarter-circular or segment of a circle, lines — single, staggered, continuous, broken and found in the iris stroma, clearly visible when pupil is narrowed. Significance disputed.

Frill: circular or cord-like formation about 1 mm away from the edge of the pupil, seldom completely round, often indented and with protrusions, variously pigmented, sometimes floating in aqueous humour, can also be wide open.

Congestion furrows: thickish, dark formations, spreading mostly outwards from the frill up to the edge of the iris, becoming thinner peripherally and with a wide base in the centre. They could also be described as long, drawn-out cone segments; can also spread out from the frill.

Lacuna: oval, superficial structural mark in the upper stroma level. Can be chambered, open or closed at the edge, occurs usually in the area of the frill.

Limbus: edge of iris.

Lipaemic: the condition of raised blood fats (hyperlipidaemia).

Lymph cords: light, but also pigmented thick, partly thinning, cordlike structures between frill and tophi. Look mostly like several radials stuck together.

Stomach definition: structural name for the stomach region.

Stomach region: peripupiliary circular zone around 1 mm wide.

Stomach ring: see stomach region.

Daisy iris: many of the flower-leaf shaped weakness marks which spread out from the frill are clearly visible in the iris stroma and reminiscent of a flower (daisy).

Mixed iris: a not entirely blue, not entirely brown iris. Iris stroma still clearly visible which is not the case in the pure brown iris. Appears mostly light brown to greenish. The mixed iris could be described as a more or less pigmented blue iris with recognisable iris stroma.

ELIMINATIVE FUNCTIONS AND ALTERATIVE CHANGES

The bowel is not an eliminative organ. The function of the alimentary tract is to absorb materials from the lumen of the gut, and this faculty extends throughout the whole length of the tract. Problems may arise if undesirable and toxic materials are taken up, either because there is no mechanism of exclusion or because the screening process has failed—either partially or completely.

The direction of movement for the absorbed material is inwards, that is, into the blood stream. There appears to be no reverse mechanism for excreting through the intestinal wall, except as some form of vicarious discharge. The material not absorbed is passed on down the tract for ultimate ejection, and because this material is very subject to putrefactive change, there must be no undue delay in its removal, otherwise degenerative products will also be absorbed.

Once in the blood, the direction of movement is into the extracellular fluids directly surrounding the tissue cells and from which unusable and waste substances are removed by the lymphatic system for ultimate elimination through the hepatic and renal functions or through the skin. Any failure or obstruction of these excretory organs will lead to an accumulation of toxic and waste matter within the tissues. It is the interstitial accumulation of metabolic residues and unusable materials which is referred to as 'encumbrance'.

This whole process is perfectly symbolised in the iris, in which the state of encumbrance is graphically portrayed. Iris illustrations 2, 24 and 26 present various degrees of this encumbrance, and the relative text discusses the formation of the appropriate iris-signs (Iris 24, see also the Introduction of Part 1).

Therapeutic objectives need to be clearly identified in each individual case if treatment is to be purposeful. Irisdiagnosis offers a depth of insight into the context of each problem otherwise unobtainable—

(1) Incomplete digestive processing and excessive permeability of the intestinal structures can be directly assessed from the indications of the gastro-intestinal zone—dark colouring, defect-signs and wreath dilatation.

(2) Disturbance of the blood and tissue fluids from absorbed

toxins and hepatic-renal dysfunction can be seen in the colour changes and pigment deposits of the second major zone.

(3) The adequacy of skin function, the level of lymphatic activity and the existence of catarrhal exudates will be shown by the indications in the peripheral zone—scurf-rim, lymphatic rosary, white clouds and flakes.

Thus zonal location identifies the sphere of dysfunction or confirms the involvement of all three in total saturation (Iris 26).

Bowel

As an absorbing organ, the large intestine takes up fluid and electrolytes, but in health screens out deleterious materials. The integrity of the mucous membrane is thus most important in problems of auto-intoxication. Although the motility of peristalsis is also a factor in deciding the duration of contact with the absorbing mucosa, the mere securing of the daily 'stool' will not affect the vulnerability of an ulcerated or over-relaxed mucous membrane.

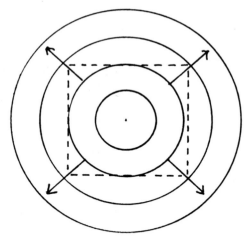

Dilatation of the wreath zone at the points of the diagonal cross, associated with stromal loosening, indicates the vulnerable locations for toxic absorption—caecum, hepatic flexure, splenic flexure and sigmoid colon (diagrammatically combining both irides). Expansion at all four locations produces the tendency to a square-shaped wreath. Such a shape has always been associated with incurable conditions and a generally poor prognosis (Iris 9/10, 47/48).

The presence of thick white bands, so-called 'lymph-bridges', extending out from the iris-wreath and terminating in peripheral white clouds, illustrate the connection between points of toxic absorption and peripheral saturation with increased lymphatic activity, note: caecum and appendix (Iris 11, 16, 19, 20), hepatic flexure (Iris 11, 12, 47), splenic flexure (5, 7, 26, 32) and sigmoid colon (5, 7, 26, 48).

These conditions so often arise in childhood from a diet containing excessive amounts of poor quality carbohydrate (white flour and sugar) and become permanently established as chronic catarrhs, often with the presence of intestinal worms. But with or without an apparent lymphatic 'rosary' or 'lymph-bridges', the wide wreath zone with signs of debility decides the principal objective in treatment: Natr.phos. for the acidity conditions produced by excessive carbohydrates, with gentle trophorestorative tonics—Agrimonia, Chelone, Juglans cin., will avoid the use of questionable anthelmintics and slowly resolve the catarrhal symptoms—subject to dietetic correction.

Caecum: Dilatation of the wreath in this area more often indicates accompanying defect-signs (Iris 11B), or deep rhomboid-signs (Iris 10E, 13A, 19H) suggesting erosion and perforation with consequent inflammatory involvement of the peritoneum and with the development of adhesions (transversals). The enclosed pocket of suppurative infection which results presents a continuing surgical hazard and provides a background for the acute appendix (Iris 11B, 19H).

It is significant that where caecal pathology has resulted from external injury, the intestinal zone does not show the deep lesions characteristic of ulcerative erosion (Iris 20B, 40C), nor the typical wreath zone dilatation. Indeed, the intestinal sign is likely to show a surrounding white ring, signifying a healed condition (Iris 40C).

Hepatic flexure: The ascending colon, including the hepatic flexure, is commonly implicated in conditions of duodenal ulceration with extensive abdominal adhesions. Iris illustrations 11C, 12D, 13, 19F and 43C, also show the wreath zone expansion and enclosed defect-signs, including wedge-signs or rhomboid-signs, as well as the peripheral white clouds and connecting white bands. Clearly, the intestinal lesions involve toxic absorption and reflex implication of the peripheral structures—in this case, the neck and ears.

It is thus not surprising to find a history of glandular congestion or catarrhal otitis when these signs are present (Iris 11, 12, 43). The response to treatment of children showing catarrhal or glandular congestion of the neck and ears will remain unsatisfactory if no attention is given to evident weakness of the colon at these locations.

Splenic flexure: Dilatation of the splenic flexure and upper part of the descending colon is most frequently related to the Roemheld syndrome. Distension of this section of the colon from flatulence obviously involves upward pressure upon the diaphragm and heart, to produce functional disturbances: palpitation, oppression, extra-systoles, etc. (Iris 9B, 26D, 30). However, Roemheld syndrome is not confined to the left side. Iris 10F shows a condition affecting the right side (hepatic flexure), producing respiratory symptoms: oppression and dyspnoea.

Illustrations 5, 7, 26 and 32, show the associated signs suggesting toxic absorption and peripheral saturation.

Sigmoid and rectum: The lower part of the descending colon and sigmoid flexure is especially subject to diverticulosis and ulcerative perforation, with consequent chronic inflammation of the peritoneum, massive adhesions (cobweb-signs) and the possible development of a gravitation abscess. Irides 7, 26 and 38, show such conditions. These illustrations also show the white clouds and 'lymph-bridges' associated with peripheral intoxication, apart from the local defect-signs. As with similar signs in the caecal area, they indicate the need for vigilance and prompt reference for surgical treatment on the appearance of acute symptoms.

Atonic states or mucosal breakdown are relatively common conditions affecting the rectum, often against a general background of connective tissue weakness and visceral prolapse. Iris illustrations 3G, 7, 26K and 30D, referring to young women, show conditions which vary from simple catarrhal discharge to haemorrhagic diarrhoea. Similar conditions in the male are less common, but an example is shown in Iris 4C, where the iris-signs are more clearly portrayed.

The objectives in treatment are to heal the mucous membrane and tone the connective tissue background, not forgetting the need to ease the superimposed pressure of any generalised visceroptosis. High rectal injections or suppositories of preparations of Calendula, Hydrastis, Capsella, Myrica, Symphytum, etc. as appropriate, together with oral calcium therapy—calc.flour., calc.phos., calc.sulph.—provide suitable medication, but in this location, response is always tardy in atonic or over-relaxed conditions.

Anus: The condition of haemorrhoids is usually associated with portal back pressure secondary to hepatic engorgement or over-contraction, but the liver itself may be subject to back pressure from cardiac insufficiency. Thus, it is not sufficient to confine the treatment of haemorrhoids to the use of local salves or suppositories. Iris illustrations 28B, 33D and 35A show conditions of venous stasis arising from cardiac weakness or pathology. As a tonic astringent to the portal veins, Collinsonia is also a mild cardiac tonic, helping to restore the normal level of blood pressure. Where blood pressure is already high from sclerotic changes, Collinsonia could be combined with Crataegus and Cimicifuga.

Prominence of ecchymoses and petechiae on the legs will indicate the systemic need for Calc.fluor. as a vascular tissue trophorestorative which will also help to control haemorrhoidal bleeding.

Iris illustrations 1H and 27J show conditions where the haemorrhoids are part of a rectal pathology. In Iris 1H, the black wedge-sign and white radial point to a lesion at a higher level of the rectum, and in Iris 27J there is a rectal tumour. Such conditions demonstrate the need to use local medication in the form of rectal injections, rather than to rely upon oral prescriptions for conditions of the lower bowel.

Kidneys

Renal competence should be assessed from simple clinical tests rather than by deducing the probable level of function from the iris-signs. Indeed, all functional activity should be so assessed. Iris indications show the long-term trophic changes from which the reserve capacity of the organ may be estimated, but the functional response can still be adequate, even when defect-signs are shown.

Three principal factors affect the ability of the kidney to excrete those metabolic end products which are sufficiently soluble to pass through the renal tubules—

(1) The organic integrity of the organ tissues (? tropho-restoratives).
(2) The blood supply to the organ (? astringents/relaxants).
(3) The functional response (? stimulants/sedatives).

The objective of medication will be to achieve optimum function by supplying an appropriate compound of physiological influences: stimulants, relaxants, astringents, demulcents, etc., as may be required. The simple clinical tests for urine concentration, water clearance, and 24-hour solids, are available to monitor the results.

Vital response: Both white and dark signs indicate functional disturbance. Acute and sub-acute inflammatory conditions (white signs) produce states of irritation and reduce the level of secretion/excretion. White signs in the kidney areas show the need for sedative influences (= soothing demulcents)—Altheae, Arctium lappa, Eryngium mar., Zea mays, etc.

Dark signs indicate a declining response—the darker the shade, the greater the decline. Such signs show the need for renal stimulants—Apium grav., Barosma, Juniperis, etc.,—strictly within the trophic capacity as indicated by the structural signs. (Decline in response in spite of stimulants raises the question of vaso-motor dysfunction or trophic insufficiency).

Organ function: The secretory function of the kidney depends upon its blood supply, as determined by the systolic level of blood pressure and the vaso-motor control of the secretory cells. Predominant over-contraction or over-relaxation produces a decline in quality or quantity of the urine, in which the kidney is unable to excrete sufficient solid wastes or water, or both. Even in the absence of local signs, general indications of sympathetic (contraction) or parasympathetic (relaxation) stress should be taken into account.

Over-relaxation produces stasis and dilatation of the organ,

172

commonly indicated in the iris showing connective-tissue weakness. Iris illustrations 1A, 6A, 16D, 18F and 43F, portray the elements to be looked for in the kidney areas—

(1) Displacement of the wreath towards the pupil in that sector (autonomic sign).
(2) The appearance of widely spaced arc-lines enclosing the sign (stasis and swelling).
(3) Loosening of the stromal texture within the arc-lines (trophic decline).

The wider the arc-lines, the greater the degree of dilatation (tumour formation = cystic hydronephrosis—Iris 34D, 45F, 46G). If the sign moves away from, rather than towards, the pupil, a condition of floating kidney or other displacement is suggested (Iris 6A, 18F, 43F).

In simple states of over-relaxation/dilatation, astringent diuretics are required, especially those favouring connective-tissue tone: Uva-ursi, Equisetum. Calc.fluor. and Silicea are indicated for the long-term treatment of a floating kidney if not submitted for surgical restoration, and may indeed produce considerable functional improvement. Extreme degrees of dilatation shown by signs with very widely spaced arc-lines appear to be characteristic of conditions due to ureteral obstruction from cystic or tumour formation (Iris 34D, 45F), for which medicinal treatment would be useless.

A temporary degree of renal over-contraction from sympathetic nervous emphasis during the first stage of a febrile reaction, probably explains the reduced and concentrated urine of the feverish patient and the need for the relaxing diuretics commonly prescribed. Otherwise, functional over-contraction may be considered as a possibility in irides which show numerous nerve-rings (asthenia/anxiety) or sectoral flattening of the pupillary margin or iris-rim (spinal viscero-somatic reflex).

Local iris-signs suggesting over-contraction lack the characteristics of dilatation-signs given above. The sclerotic changes indicated in irides 15E, 24B and 26H (long black signs), suggest a background of over-contraction (see Organ Inferiorities), and show the need for relaxing diuretics: Capsella, Eupatorium purp., Galium, Sambucus nig., etc., which are also valuable to counter possible stone formation arising from concentration of the secretions. In these conditions, diuretic agents are best given as infusions or decoctions to secure a solvent action. Sodium and magnesium salts in low potency are indicated for sclerotic degeneration.

Peripheral encumbrance

Connective tissues not only serve as structural support, but provide a matrix for certain chemical buffer reactions and accommodate the interstitial deposition of substances not cleared from the tissues. Systemic encumbrance from endotoxicosis and exotoxicosis consists largely of such interstitial deposits.

The zones of the iris represent the tissues from centre to periphery. The deposition of waste products not fully eliminated takes place first in the peripheral tissues, especially the subcutaneous connective tissue. Deposition will be in accordance with local circulatory activity. Therefore, it is to be expected that in the skeletal system, chronic accumulations occur in and around joints and ultimately give rise to various degrees of arthritis.

As the darker shade of the outer rings extends inwards towards the pupil, so the person moves progressively away from living function towards central decline and death. The heavy, thick black scurf-rim is a sign of impending death, and any local area change towards darker colouring indicates a declining vital function to the point of necrosis and tissue destruction (deep black signs). Iris illustrations 16, 2, 23, 29 and 56, viewed in that order, show this progressive toxic saturation.

Apart from a poorly balanced diet containing excessive carbohydrates, the two principal causes of auto-intoxication are—

(1) absorption of putrefactive materials from a faulty bowel, and
(2) some degree of renal failure.

With such conditions, the organism promotes elimination through the skin and mucous membranes:

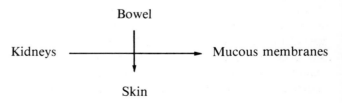

174

Mucous membranes, especially those of the upper respiratory passages, naso-pharynx and bronchi, offer a large surface area in which a normal mucous secretion serves to carry off those waste materials able to transude through the membrane and thus become a channel of vicarious excretion. All catarrhal discharges indicate a local or general form of elimination. The membranes of the rectum and vagina also serve a similar purpose.

Substances which are not able to pass through the mucous membranes (probably large or complex molecules) must be removed through the skin in the form of eruptions—acne vulgaris, furunculosis, etc., where suppuration is involved. Absorption of unreduced foreign proteins through an ulcerated or permeable gut surface provides the basis for allergic skin reactions and eczematous conditions.

The capacity of both skin and mucous membranes to function as eliminative organs is limited. In any case, catarrhal and eruptive conditions are often suppressed by local applications and drugs, so that systemic encumbrance progressively increases. The early degree evident in Iris 1, where the good skin function is able to compensate for the weak bowel, increases to that shown in Iris 3, where the thicker scurf-rim and peripheral white flakes and clouds indicate reduced skin elimination and increased susceptibility to catarrhal colds.

For so long as there is good lymphatic function, as shown by the peripheral circle of white flakes (= lymphatic rosary—see Iris 3), there will be good resistance. But the inward deviation (Iris 49A) and final disappearance of these signs, or even worse, the appearance of dark-black points (Iris 28, 29) show that lymphatic action is defunct and the scene set for purulent decomposition (Iris 55).

Providing the white clouds or radials extend to the outer iris-rim (Iris 26, 32, 43), elimination will extend through skin eruptions and the internal condition be relieved. Consequently, local treatment of eczema is not without danger if the internal causes are neglected. Continued disparity between absorption and excretion must lead to progressive accumulation and, in the absence of any form of vicarious elimination, the peripheral encumbrance produces rheumatic symptoms and developing arthritis. That these symptoms vary with the level of transudation through the skin is readily apparent in the reaction to wet weather. Suppression of catarrhal exudations will likewise aggravate arthritic tendencies (Iris 8, 15, 17, 34).

Medication and treatment

The formulation of a medicinal prescription seeks to achieve two objectives:

(1) To counter the patho-physiological influences which have contributed to the presenting conditions, and
(2) To provide forces of positive recovery for the functions and tissues involved.

Failure to achieve the first objective implies that recovery is obstructed and relapse is certain. Thus, failure to adjust the diet, or to counter the effects of psychosomatic stress, or to discontinue damaging drugs, will offset or neutralise the constructive forces available from medicines.

Medication for problems of elimination or auto-intoxication, including skin eruptions, catarrhal discharges and rheumatic syndromes, will need to cover the following aspects—

(1) Content and balance of the diet.
(2) The autonomic background to functional disturbance.
(3) Over-contracted or over-relaxed state of the intestinal tract.
(4) Permeability of the intestinal mucous membranes, i.e. structural lesions.
(5) Disturbed intermediate metabolism—liver, pancreas, kidneys.
(6) Renal excretion.
(7) The activity of the lymphatic system.
(8) Vicarious excretion from mucous membranes or skin— eruptions and catarrhal discharges.

The acid-base balance of the diet is fundamental to conditions of encumbrance. Dietetic adjustment alone will be sufficient where organ integrity is sound and functional imbalance is minimal. Unhappily, the situation is usually more complex, but even so, an adjustment of the diet to provide a predominance of fruit and vegetables with minimal starches, fats and proteins, will gradually secure the alkaline effect required. Other considerations must decide whether to use diet as a specific eliminative technique —monodiets, restrictive diets, fasting, etc.

Autonomic imbalance is more often a background consideration than an immediate objective and is usually the expression of psychosomatic stress or typological bias. However, typical vagotonic symptoms, such as excessive motility (diarrhoea), mucous colitis, or spastic constipation, in patients showing a small pupil, contracted wreath and radii solaris, will require the inclusion of a suitable nervine relaxant in the prescription: Mag.phos., Dioscorea, Matricaria, Spiraea, Viburnum, etc. Similarly, anxiety-based reactions (sympatheticotonic), intestinal colics and sphincter spasms, in patients with dilated pupils and numerous nerve rings, indicate the need for appropriate nervines: Kali phos., Pulsatilla, Lycopus, Caulophyllum, etc.

It is not for long that a functional over-contraction or over-relaxation of the intestine can exist without trophic changes taking place. Continued over-contraction of the organ tissues will lead to induration and atrophy, with darker colour and pigment deposits appearing in the iris. Protracted over-relaxation will produce tissue laxity and swelling, showing textural looseness in the gastro-intestinal zone of the iris. Thus, in the adult it becomes a question of relaxing or toning trophorestoratives rather than the simple relaxants or tonics useful in young children with intestinal symptoms—Matricaria, Pulsatilla, Agrimonia, Populus, Rubus id., Spiraea, etc. Typical trophorestorative remedies for adult problems are: Relaxing—Chelidonium, Chionanthes, Dioscorea, Leptandra; Toning—Berberis, Collinsonia, Hydrastis, Juglans. Medication for the colon is best if administered in the form of capsules or tablets to avoid affecting the alimentary function adversely. Liquid preparations for the colon are better given by rectum, especially if powerful astringency is needed.

More severe conditions (defect-signs with lymph-bridges) require powerful astringent-tonics or tonics with astringents—Juglans, Hamamelis, Hydrastis, Geranium, Symphytum, etc.—for ulceration and/or haemorrhagic discharge. Where iris-signs suggest intestinal perforation or diverticulosis, Echinacea or Baptisia is added. These medicines are best administered per rectum for maximum effect on the colon and minimal upset to the stomach. If the lesions are fairly low in the rectum, lactose-based suppositories may be effective. Appropriate biochemic salts are given for the tissue conditions—Calc.fluor., Calc.phos., Calc.sulph., Kali sulph.—to restore membrane integrity.

Metabolic disturbances show colour changes and pigment deposits in the iris, especially in the third minor zone (blood and vital fluids). A diffused translucent yellow colour around the iris-wreath suggests disturbance of renal function, whereas yellow-ochre/brown flakes or granules ('tobacco-snuff' pigment) indicate involvement of liver function. Orange pigments suggest pancreatic dysfunction, while a dirty-yellow change in the colour of the white flakes around the iris-wreath suggests gouty degeneration (See T. Kriege: *Fundamental Basis of Irisdiagnosis*). Alterative medication for the indicated organ disturbance is included in the prescription compound.

Skin eruptions or catarrhal discharges should be neither encouraged nor suppressed. These vital but vicarious reactions will subside when the basic causes are treated. Being much more frequently found in children, especially those fed on dried milk and starches, they usually respond well to biochemic treatment—Natr.phos., Kali mur., Kali sulph.—after radical adjustment of feeding. Old foci of suppressed catarrhs in the adult pose a much more dangerous problem. Chronic conditions of the ears and sinuses need very careful handling to avoid a toxaemic backlash (see Iris 12 as an example of a potentially dangerous situation).

Irisdiagnosis in rheumatic disease clearly identifies the major problem—intestinal absorption, hepatic-renal dysfunction, suppressed skin activity, focal infection, etc.—and indicates the best line of approach to a complex problem.

CIRCULATORY AND NERVOUS EQUILIBRIUM

Iris-signs consist of reflexes of autonomic origin depicting vegetative conditions. Consequently, the iris provides minimal direct information concerning the peripheral circulatory system or the central nervous system. However, some useful information may be derived from the indications of the organ areas and the zonal colour distribution.

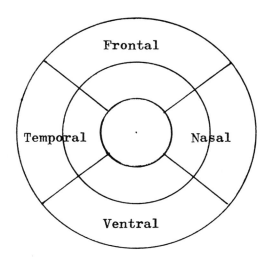

Circulatory

The regional distribution of the blood depends entirely upon effective vaso-motor control to ensure that increased supply to one part (vaso-relaxation) is balanced by reduction to another (vaso-contraction). Chronic pooling of the blood in some part of the vascular bed, due to over-relaxed tissue conditions, implies the existence of a functional ischaemia elsewhere, and with the influence of gravity, it is the cerebral supply which suffers insufficiency and the splanchnic distribution which is subject to engorgement.

Three potential conditions of chronic imbalance should always be reviewed: cerebral/splanchnic, cerebral/peripheral and visceral/peripheral. Since chronic ischaemia produces subfunction and long-term decline, then to note the distribution of the light and dark areas in the iris as between the inner and outer zones and the frontal and ventral quadrants, is to derive information concerning circulatory activity. Iris illustrations 4, 41, 47 and 51, show conditions in which an increased area of dark colouring in the frontal quadrant (brain) is opposite to light areas in the ventral quadrant (pelvic organs), suggesting that chronic hyperaemia in the pelvis has resulted in cerebral ischaemia. The relevant conditions are discussed in the text.

The existence of a bluish arc on the sclera immediately adjacent to the border in the frontal quadrant also signifies ischaemia and is a common finding in patients with low blood pressure, especially those of asthenic constitution. If this sign is accompanied by signs of relaxation in the splanchnic distribution or the extremities (visceroptosis, varicosities, leg swelling, etc., or a wide wreath-zone in the ventral quadrant of the iris) then it is clear that medication is needed to restore the balance. Collinsonia or Myrica to contract the lower vascular channels, together with Betonica to increase supply to the head, will improve depressive headaches or other functional disturbances. This possibility should be remembered with vertex headaches occurring during menstruation.

A comparable situation is found in the patient with pallid skin and flabby tissues, where the wide dark scurf-rim represents the peripheral vascular stasis. In this case, the Betonica for the head circulation needs to be combined with Myrica for the peripheral relaxation and Xanthoxylum for the low systolic level.

The appearance of arcs and rings in the outer zones indicates various forms of sclerotic change. The arcus senilis (Iris-25) is expected in old age, but has a more ominous prognosis in the earlier years (Iris 13). The 'sodium'-ring (American terminology) or 'cholesterol'-ring (German terminology) may or may not have anything to do with the excessive ingestion of table salt or fats. A sclerotic arc in the brain area is certainly a feature of arteriosclerosis or ischaemic induration and may also indicate metallic poisoning (Iris 5, 31, 35). Whatever the aetiology, the sign indicates more difficult transudation of fluids and the need for softening and resolvent medicinal influences: Natr.mur., Mag.phos., Betonica, Cimicifuga, Scutellaria, Urtica, etc. Meanwhile, tissue nutrition requires a somewhat higher systolic level where possible to improve function.

The combination of a very dark outer zone with a bright white inner zone shows visceral irritation from internal congestion (Iris 2, 23). Marked regional increase in the width of the scurf-rim in the temporal quadrants: Right iris—lungs and liver; Left iris—lungs and spleen, indicates local chronic congestion (Iris 16, 26, 28, 38). If the iris also shows a displacement of the lymphatic flakes inwards towards the pupil (Iris 22, 24, 40) a suppressed or unresolved pathology is likely. The more the dark colouring moves inwards, the less favourable the prognosis, either general or local.

Nervous

Pupillary function reflects the dual control of the autonomic nervous system. Dilatation of the pupil is activated by sympathetic nerve impulses and contraction results from parasympathetic action. A tendency for the pupil to remain unduly dilated is usually due to excessive sympathetic activity. Similarly, marked over-contraction of the pupil results from increased parasympathetic activity or irritation. Constant or predominant dilatation probably explains the formation of nerve-rings, whereas prolonged contraction produces a congestive bunching of the radial fibres of the inner zones and the formation of radii solaris. Thus:

Nerve rings = sympatheticotonia = asthenic response = Ca need.
Radii solaris = vagotonia = hypersthenic response = Mg need.

These broad indications can decide the choice of medication for the background to whatever condition is presented. Thus:

(1) Asthenic syndromes (sympathetic stress)—nervine tonics and trophorestoratives.
(2) Hypersthenic syndromes (parasympathetic stress)—relaxing nervines and pure relaxants.

The presence of numerous nerve rings will suggest the use of nervine tonics such as—Pulsatilla, Scutellaria, Valeriana, whereas radii solaris indicate the need for—Cypripedium, Dioscorea, Matricaria, etc. The extreme conditions suggested by the presence of both nerve rings and radii solaris, especially when chronic and deeply scored in the haematogenous iris-constitution (spasm-ophilia), usually respond well to such powerful nervine antispasmodics as: Valeriana + Viburnum opulus.

ORGAN INFERIORITIES

Insufficient functional capacity, an organ 'inferiority', may arise from various causes:

(1) genetic weakness or restricted development,
(2) permanent damage from previous illness or injury,
(3) destructive pathological processes—infective, tubercular, toxic or malignant,
(4) Progressive deterioration from defective blood and nerve supply—fatty degeneration, simply atrophy, fibrotic or sclerotic change.

Permanent weakness, whether genetic, developmental or acquired, where there is no continuing pathology or progressive decline, is usually shown by a closed lacuna in the organ area. Although the reserve capacity is limited, there will be no symptoms of stress providing the life-style makes no excessive demand upon that function. Treatment is not required, although the incapacity must be considered in the general prognosis.

Destructive pathological processes are systemic and to be treated as such. There are no pathognomonic iris-signs to indicate the origin of the pathology, although skilled interpretation of a number of signs taken together may establish the probable cause. The signs available show the extent of tissue destruction together with the associated indications of vital reactivity and resistance. Hence, tubercular and malignant conditions will often show a mixture of white and black signs (see the series of tubercular conditions illustrated in Irides 43-52).

Progressive deterioration involving retrograde tissue change, atrophic or sclerotic, arises from dysfunction in which the nutrition of the organ is disturbed by over-contraction (ischaemia) or over-relaxation (stasis). Such conditions are theoretically reversible short of essential cell destruction.

There are two quite distinct routes of pathological deterioration:

(1) Over-contraction = ischaemia ⟶ increased deposits of waste and toxic residues ⟶ fibrotic/sclerotic degeneration.
(2) Over-relaxation = overhydration ⟶ local stasis and congestion ⟶ atrophic degeneration.

In the former condition of dehydration-degeneration-induration, the iris signs consist of white signs declining to dark clouds and wisps, with ultimate development of penetrating defect-signs, showing the need for stimulating alteratives and relaxing trophorestoratives. In the latter condition of dilatation-stasis-atrophy, the signs consist of wide separation of the radial fibres with the appearance of dark colouring between, typically seen within the arc-lines of an open lacuna. The medicinal influences required are astringent trophorestoratives and connective tissue tonics.

Brain

The brain is the organ of the mind. As an instrument of perception and volition it serves the function of the personality, and as with all other organs, it will be affected by the same influences which determine functional efficiency and organic integrity.

Many mental and psychological symptoms do not have their origin in the mind but result from deficient blood supply. Psychotherapy is pointless when feelings of anxiety arise from deficient cerebral circulation and nutrition. The asthenic patient with numerous nerve rings will be much less distressed when calcium and potassium activity is improved (Calc.phos., Kali phos.). Likewise the deep cerebral fatigue suggested by dark radii solaris in the frontal quadrant.

In the nature of the upright position, the head organs suffer more than other parts of the body from deficient blood supply (dark colour, blue scleral rim in the upper iris quadrant). Depressive or melancholic symptoms far more often need influences to transfer the blood from elsewhere—Betonica with Collinsonia/Myrica, together with Xanthoxylum if an arterial tonic influence is needed (Iris 6E). If general tissue laxity is evident, positive trophorestorative nervines are indicated—Valeriana, Scutellaria; especially those which also have a supportive action on the alimentary processes—Rosmarinus, Humulus, Carduus bened. (Iris 16G, 27G, 47E). The reputation of Betonica, Rosmarinus and Carduus, for poor memory and deficient recall rests upon their tonic and trophic actions.

Cardiac lesions obviously affect peripheral circulation and the head is most vulnerable. The frontal sclerotic arc is the earliest sign in arteriosclerosis (Iris-33F). Spinal injury affects the neck to produce cerebral vaso-constriction and circulatory obstruction (Iris 36J). Such involvement from remote lesions needs medicinal influences to counter the effects when head symptoms develop: Scutellaria and Pulsatilla to relax the cerebral circulation, with Cimicifuga for sclerotic degeneration.

Heart

The principal signs indicating some degree of cardiac insufficiency, however slight or clinically unconfirmed, are lacunae and defect-signs. Lacunae, whether open or closed, indicate weakness, and may contain defect-signs to indicate tissue damage, either progressive or resolved. The open lacuna is primarily a connective tissue sign and in the heart area suggests potential dilatation in which the integrity of the supportive tissue is weakened (Iris 31C). Since the apposition of the valve cusps and the effectiveness of contractile action depends upon the connective tissue background, medicinal action is primarily directed to supporting these tissues: Calc.fluor., Calc.phos., Silicea, Myrica, Collinsonia, Populus, etc., are the effective influences needed in the typically atonic post-febrile condition.

Deterioration is seen in the loss of radial fibre regularity within the arms of the lacuna—darkening and separation of fibres (Iris 39), honeycomb formation (Iris 32), defect-signs, torpedo- or rhomboid-signs (Iris 33, 34, 35). Defect-signs close to the iris-wreath suggest valve damage, whereas those further out show lesions of the myocardium (infarct). The immediate prognosis is obviously related to the extent of organic damage, in which the depth and extent of defect-signs is the measure. The objectives in treatment are to reduce functional demands to within the available capacity and to provide trophorestorative influences: Kali phos., Calc.phos., Convallaria, Crataegus.

Depending upon the general background, further deterioration shows two main divisions—

(1) atrophic = dilatation and incompetence (Iris 31, 39),
(2) sclerotic = enlargement and induration (Iris 33, 35)

Medication for atrophic conditions needs to be restorative and supportive: Cereus/Convallaria with Myrica/Collinsonia,

Calc.fluor./Calc.phos., whereas that for sclerotic degeneration is resolvent and relaxant: Crataegus, Cimicifuga, Ballota, Phytolacca, Mag.phos., Kali phos.

Subsidiary considerations require the addition of auxiliary influences to the compound prescription:

(1) Spiraea with suitable alteratives and diuretics for a rheumatic background. Natr.phos. (Chalky-blue iris—Iris 34).
(2) Echinacea and Calendula for focal infection (Iris 30).
(3) Ballota for coronary spasm and angina. Mag.phos. (Iris 33).
(4) Matricaria or Pulsatilla for organ neurosis—'anger' or anxiety. Mag.phos./Kali phos. (Iris 31).

Traditionally, the closed lacuna suggests a resolved condition in which compensation has been established, although reserve capacity is usually diminished. The iris will often show signs indicating that some acute cardiac condition has existed, from which the patient has recovered (Iris 3, 37). Although treatment as such is not considered necessary, yet positive medicinal support may be indicated where the weakened heart is likely to be exposed to increased stress. In spite of voluntary control of behaviour, in order to remain within the existing cardiac capacity, the demands of a febrile reaction could break down the compensation and so produce an acute crisis—especially in children (Iris 32). Moreover, the evidence of a previously resolved condition (closed lacuna) does not prevent deterioration from current stress (Iris 40) or from gradual sclerotic change (Iris 38).

Lungs and Bronchi

The mucous membrane of the upper respiratory tract provides a large surface area for the vicarious elimination of waste substances in the form of catarrhal discharges. The degenerative conditions resulting from chronic catarrh account for the majority of diseases affecting the naso-pharynx and bronchi. It is the suppressive treatment of such conditions during childhood which paves the way for chronic sinusitis, otitis, bronchitis and catarrhal asthma in the adult years.

The cause of all catarrhal discharges lies in the disparity between the accumulation and elimination of waste products, in which faulty diet, toxic absorption, renal insufficiency and inadequate skin function participate. Repeated colds and coughs in children are the signal to review these possible causes and to look for the appropriate signs in the iris. The principles of medication discussed under 'Eliminative Functions and Alterative Changes' apply to most of the typical clinical conditions.

Chronic pulmonary disease in the adult consists largely of unresolved or suppressed conditions together with atrophic and degenerative tissue changes. The two lacunae shown in the pulmonary areas of Iris 21 are immediately apparent, as is the much darker pulmonary sector of Iris 24. The same sector of Iris 20 is less striking, but closer examination shows greater disruption of the radial structure and the presence of numerous defect-signs. A wider dark scurf-rim, together with the inward movement of lymphatic signs (Iris 20, 24) suggests that previous conditions have been suppressed. In these patients the conditions are mainly due to gastro-intestinal dysfunction and mal-absorption. Signs for chronic renal involvement are also seen.

Catarrhal discharges should be neither encouraged nor suppressed, they will diminish when the body has no further need for them. But chronic conditions ultimately produce over-relaxation and debility of the mucous membranes, indicating the need for tonic-astringent influences in treatment for trophic recovery. The choice of medicines must avoid both powerfully stimulating and strongly astringent substances, selecting those agents which achieve resolution without upsetting or disturbing reactions. Inula, Sticta and Symphytum, are suitable trophorestoratives, especially in the elderly. Prunus virg. may be added for chronic bronchial irritability, Solidago for putrescent discharges, Lycopus virg. for haemoptysis, etc.

Catarrhal debility in children results in the development of a croupy cough, especially in those showing nerve rings in the iris. A compound of Trifolium, Sambucus and Hyssopus, together with Scutellaria or Hypericum as a nervine tonic, will prove effective. Calcium salts should always be prescribed for children showing nerve rings, and alternating Kali mur./Kali sulph. for the catarrhal discharge.

Naso-pharyngeal catarrh with chronic sinusitis or otitis is a potentially dangerous condition at any age. The development of a wedge-sign in the iris organ area is an indication of chronicity, especially when the point of the wedge penetrates the iris-wreath to show autonomic involvement (Iris 12—very obvious. Iris 6, 16, 24.). These conditions often rest upon a background of hereditary tuberculosis (Iris 11, 13), or have a history of asthma or pertussis (Iris 16, 40). According to Theodor Kriege, unresolved or suppressed pulmonary conditions are responsible for the persistence of chronic naso-pharyngeal disease. These underlying influences may require skilled homoeopathic techniques (nosodes) to help resolve the clinical symptoms. All of the iris illustrations referred to show kidney signs and/or pleural adhesions, and in all cases the prognosis is poor.

Secretory organs

The functions of the principal secretory organs—liver, pancreas and kidneys—have been discussed in relation to alimentation and elimination. Since their secretions are conveyed by ducts, the organs are vulnerable to congestion and back pressure when obstructive conditions restrict the onward flow of the secretions, leading to dilatation and swelling of the organ affected. Thus, duodenal constriction with scar tissue formation and adhesions produces back pressure on the liver and gall-bladder, or on the pancreas (Iris 12D). Similarly, ureteral obstruction from the outside pressure of pelvic tumours or adhesions affects renal excretion and produces dilatation and hydronephrosis (Iris 41L). Such conditions are frankly surgical and are recognised by the excessive width of the sign (= tumour-sign).

The restoration of increased functional capacity in a secretory organ depends upon stimulating sufficient trophic activity and improving the blood supply. Trophorestorative remedies combine a gentle degree of relaxation with mild sustained stimulation, so that the optimum conditions for recovery are provided without disturbing function. However, where the local conditions are excessively contracted or already over-relaxed to the point of stasis, then adjunctive influences may be necessary as relaxants or tonics accordingly.

Thus, in the treatment of the kidneys, Verbena or Capsella provide a combination of qualities suitable for long-term use. The choice of one or other, according to the need for slight relaxation or astringency, could be supported by Galium or Caulophyllum to provide even greater relaxation (Iris 15), or with Agrimonia or Uva-ursi for more tonic-astringency (Iris 19). Where a floating kidney is shown in the context of connective-tissue weakness (Iris 6, 18), appropriate astringent-tonics are needed: Equisetum, Uva-ursi, Ruta graveolens.

The secretions of the liver and pancreas flow to the duodenum and are involved in digestive processes. The trophic background to these functions is interpreted mainly from the iris-signs seen in the temporal quadrant of the right iris in the second and third minor zones, where the structures may be considerably distorted (Iris 12, 18). In this sector, the overall texture of the wreath zone and the contraction or dilatation of the iris-wreath indicate the major influence required, either relaxing or contracting, while the local defect-signs show the extent of organic deterioration and give some idea of the likely response. The presence of extensive adhesions (Iris 6, 12), defect-signs (Iris 16, 19), or signs of induration (Iris 17, 25) give little hope of improvement.

Suitable trophorestorative agents for the liver, duodenum and pancreas, are: Chelidonium—mildly relaxing, and Chionanthes —gentle bitter tonic. The addition of Dioscorea for greater relaxation, or Berberis vulg., to increase tonicity, with Iris vers. as the suitable alterative, extends the medicinal influence. Long-term low-level dosage is indicated and a tablet or pill form is preferable. However, trophic recovery of the upper abdominal organs depends very greatly upon normalising the costal and diaphragmatic components of breathing, in order to improve circulation through the liver and to release tension of the solar plexus. Neither the asthenic constitution with retracted diaphragm and scaphoid abdomen, nor the hypersthenic habitus with barrel chest and abdominal ptosis, can be expected to respond to medication alone.

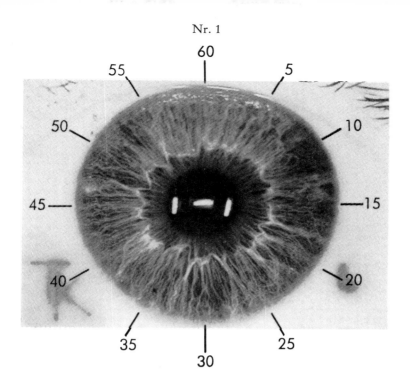

Nr. 1

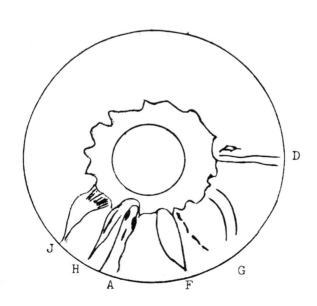

Iris 1—left

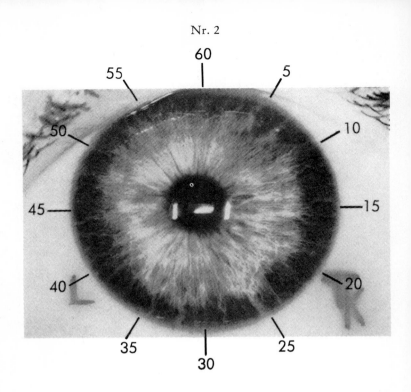

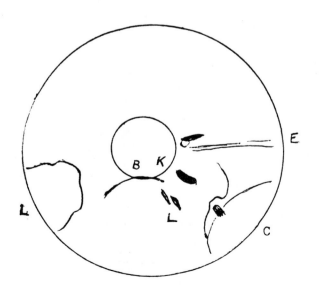

Iris 2—left

Nr. 3

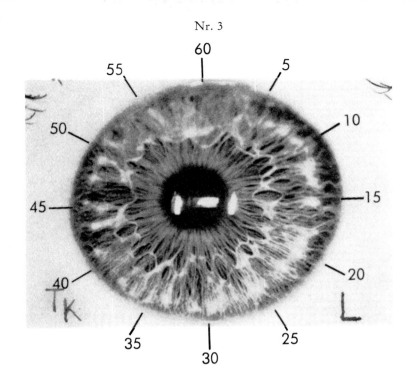

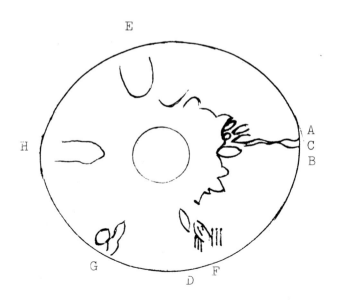

Iris 3—left

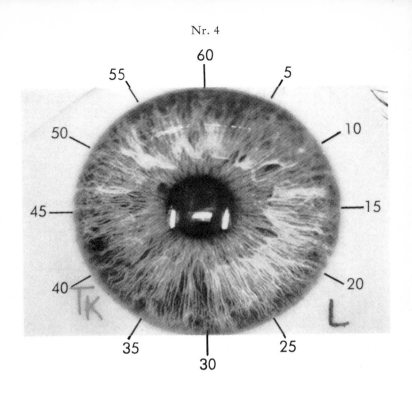

Nr. 4

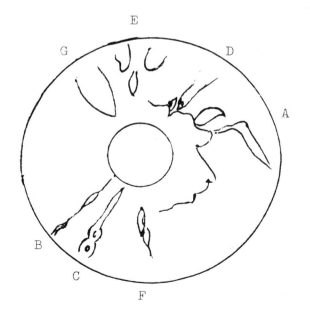

Iris 4—left

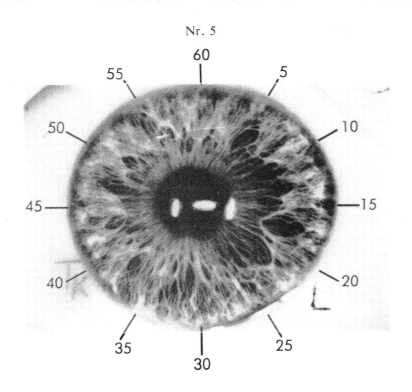

Nr. 5

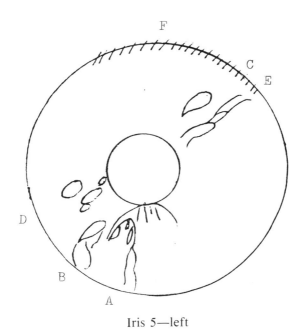

Iris 5—left

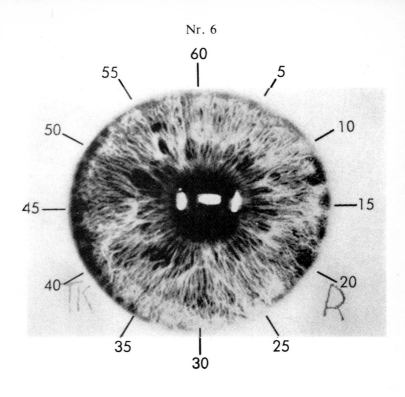

Nr. 6

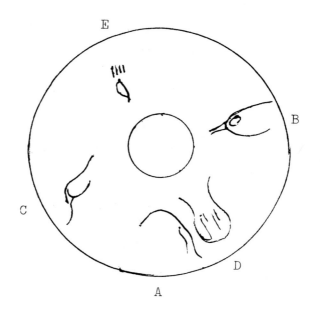

Iris 6—right

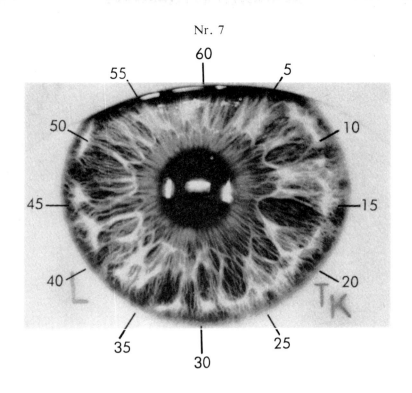

Nr. 7

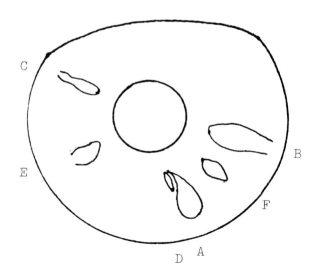

Iris 7—left

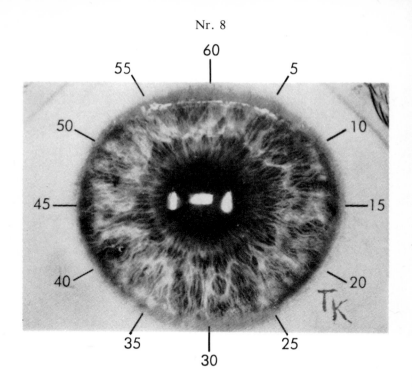

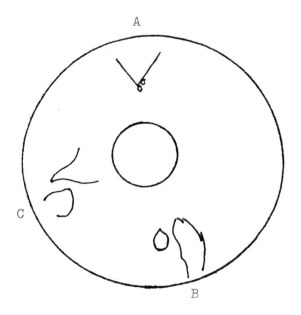

Iris 8—left

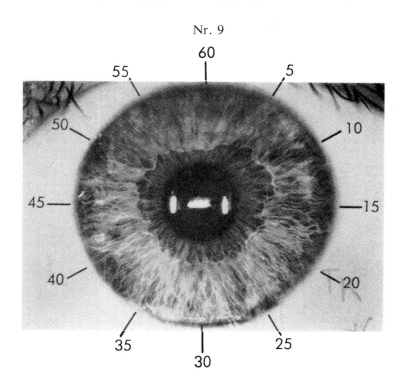

Nr. 9

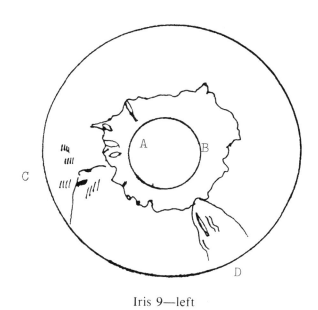

Iris 9—left

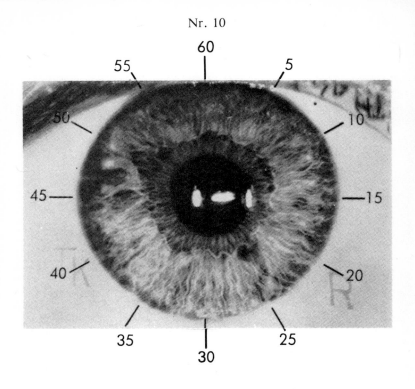

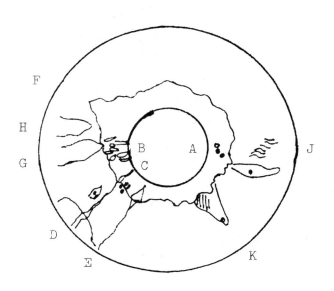

Iris 10—right

Nr. 11

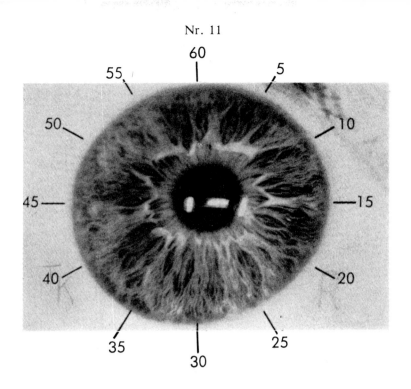

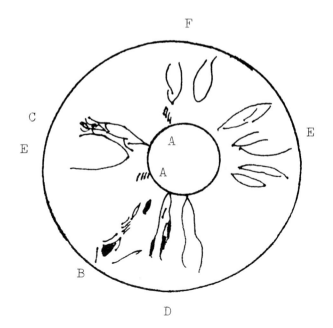

Iris 11—right

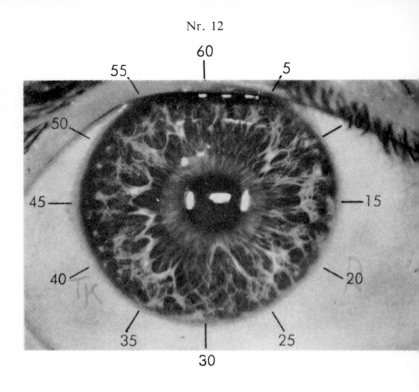

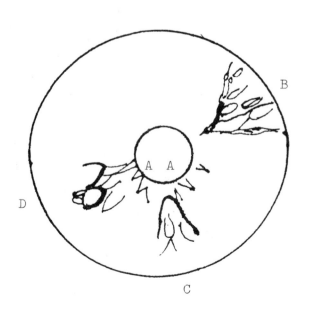

Iris 12—right

Nr. 13

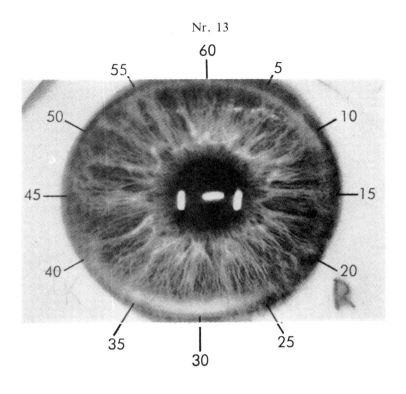

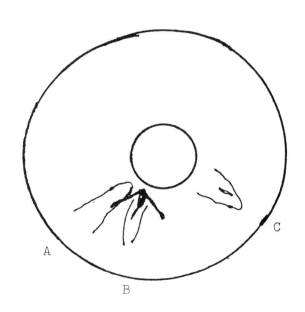

Iris 13—right

Nr. 14

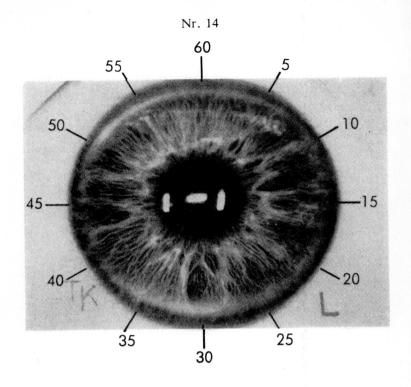

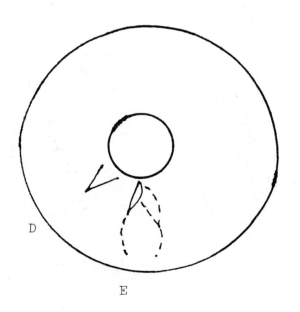

Iris 14—left

202

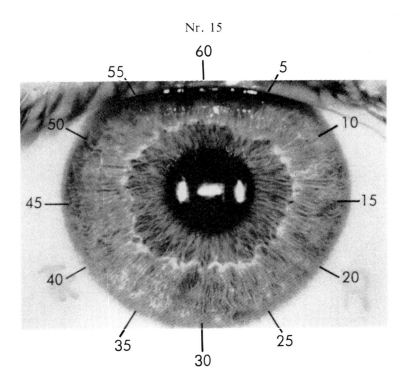

Nr. 15

60
55
5
50
10
45
15
40
20
35
25
30

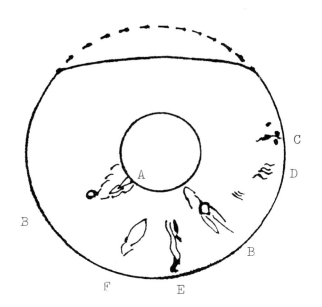

A
B
C
D
B
F
E

Iris 15—right

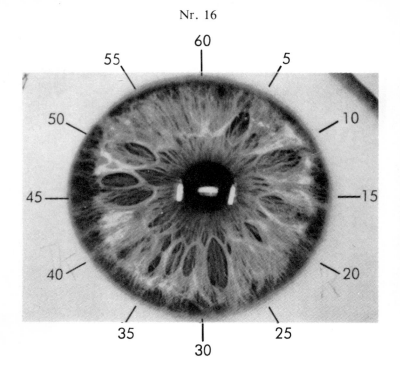

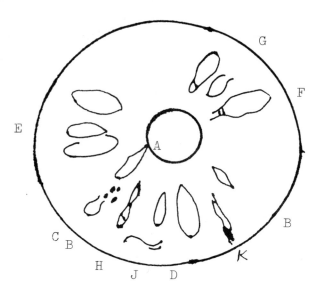

Iris 16—right

Nr. 17

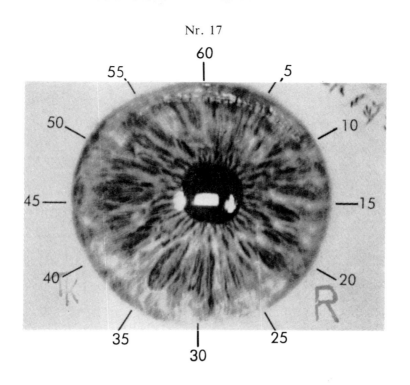

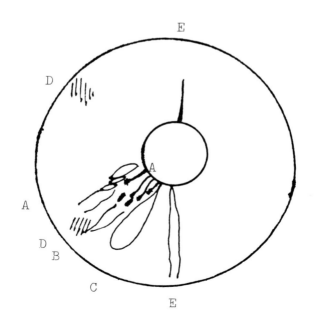

Iris 17—right

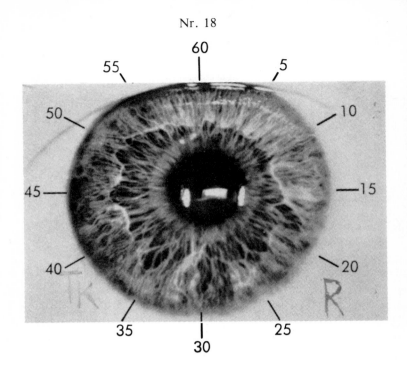

Nr. 18

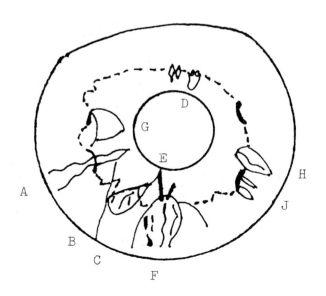

Iris 18—right

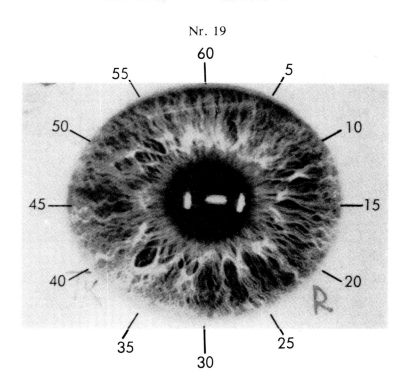

Nr. 19

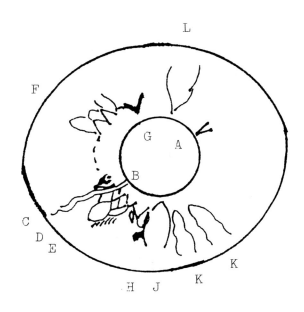

Iris 19—right

Nr. 20

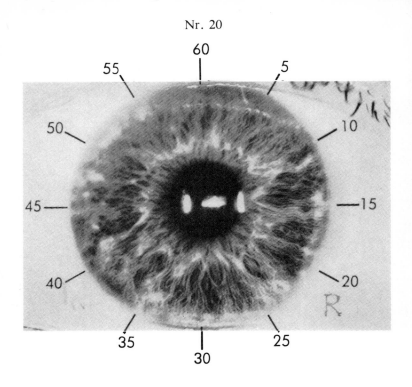

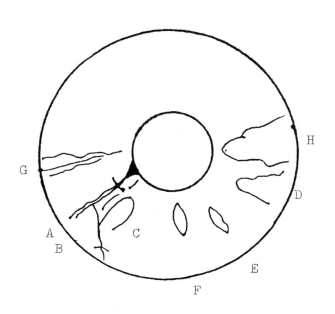

Iris 20—right

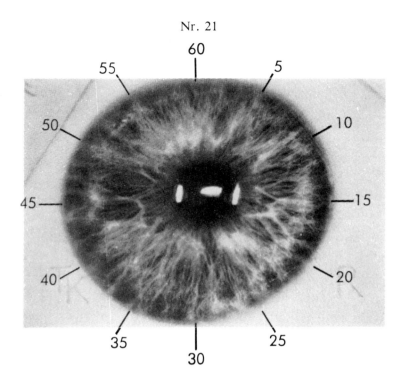

Nr. 21

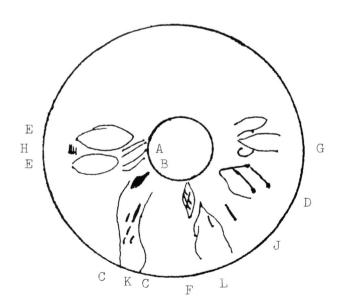

Iris 21—right

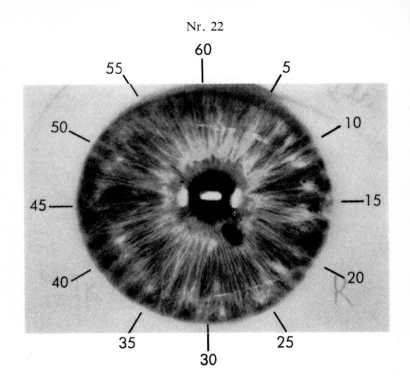

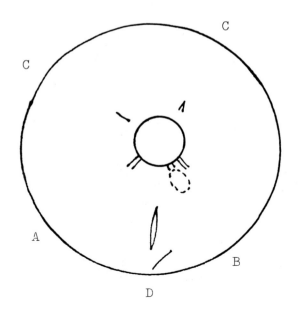

Iris 22—right

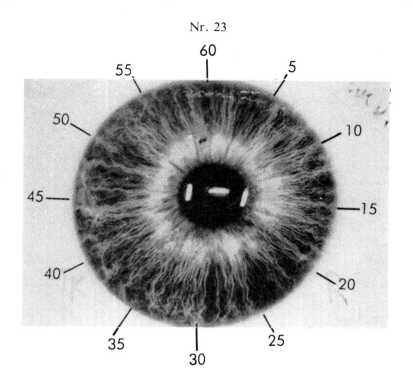

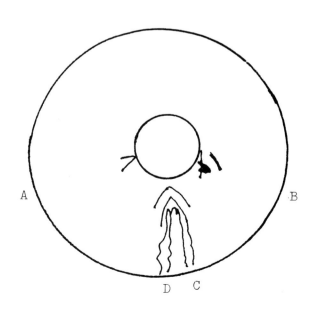

Iris 23—right

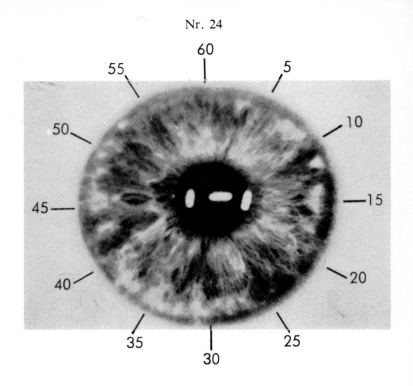

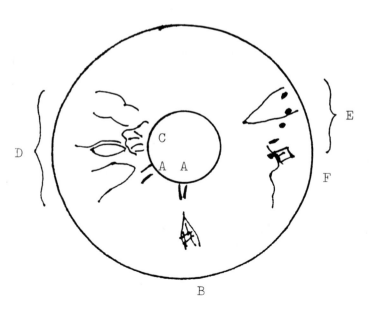

Iris 24—right

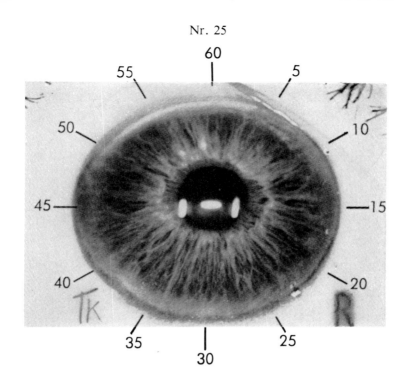

Nr. 25

60
55
5
50
10
45
15
40
20
35
25
30

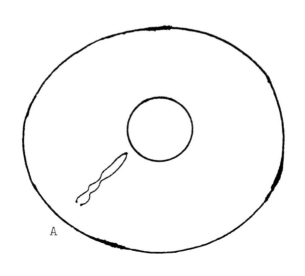

A

Iris 25—right

Nr. 26

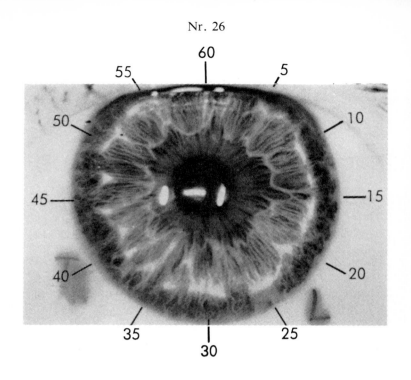

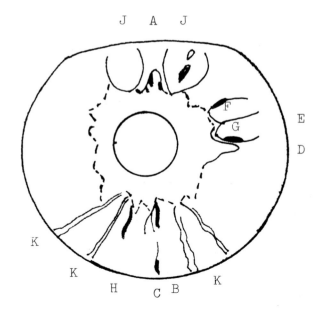

Iris 26—left

Nr. 26

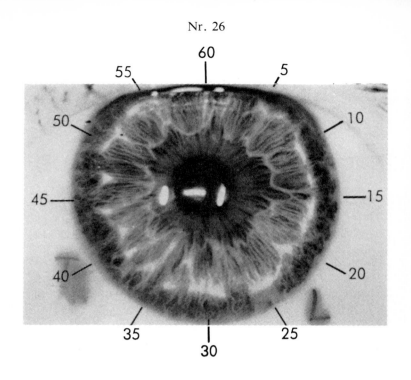

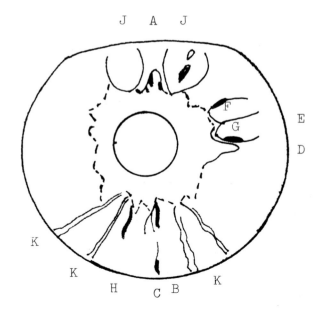

Iris 26—left

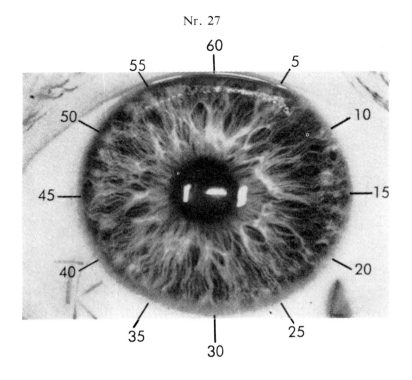

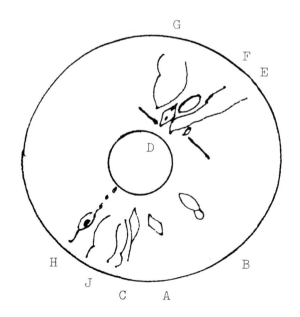

Iris 27—left

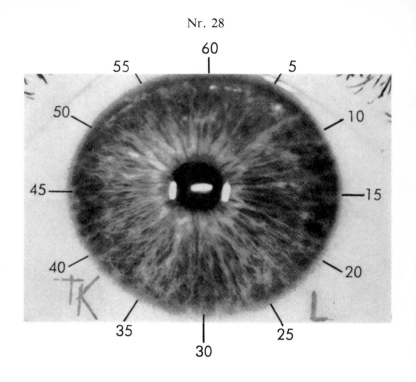

Nr. 28

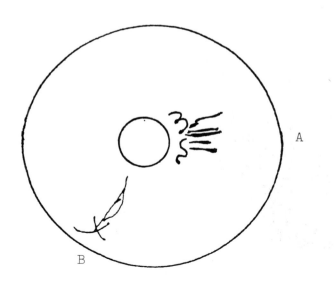

Iris 28—left

Nr. 29

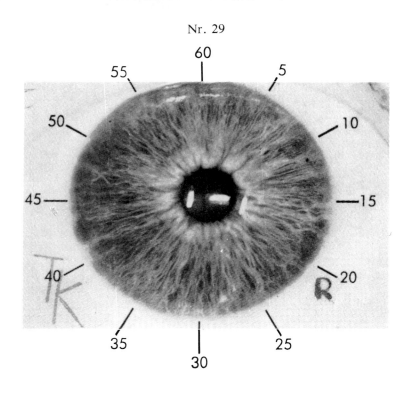

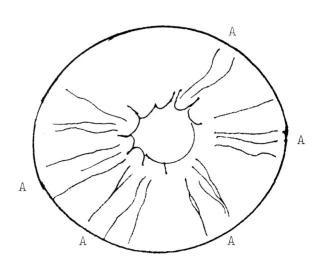

Iris 29—right

Nr. 30

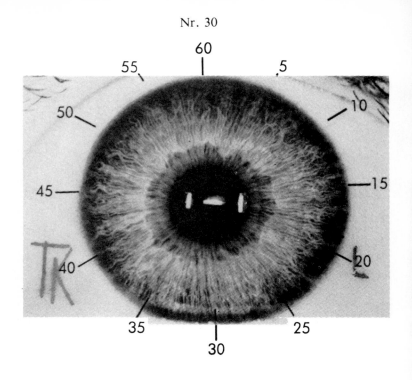

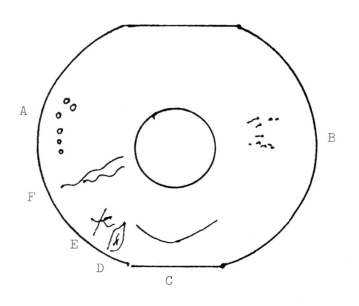

Iris 30—left

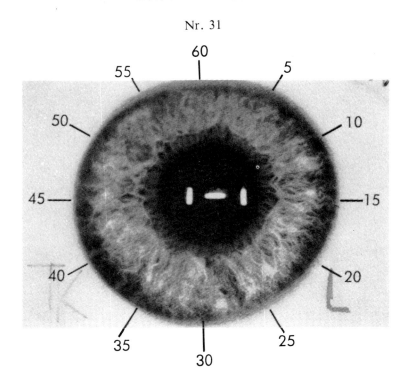

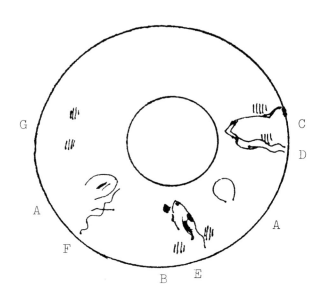

Iris 31—left

Nr. 32

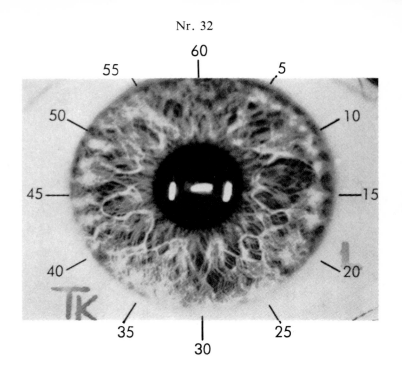

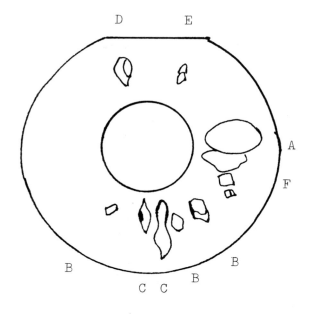

Iris 32—left

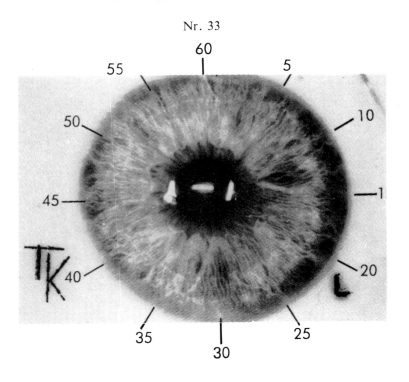

Nr. 33

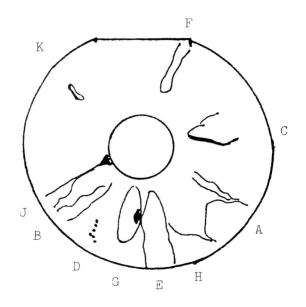

Iris 33—left

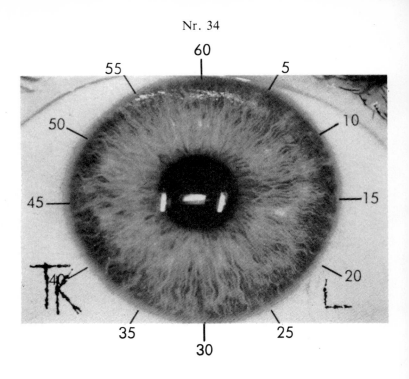

Nr. 34

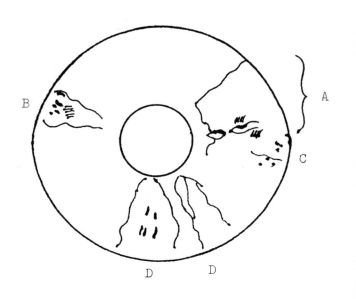

Iris 34—left

Nr. 35

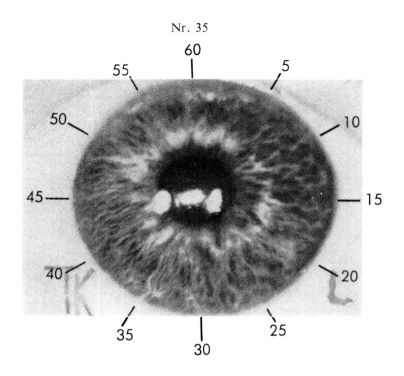

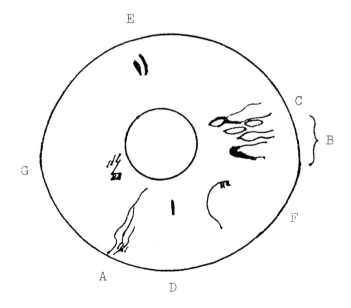

Iris 35—left

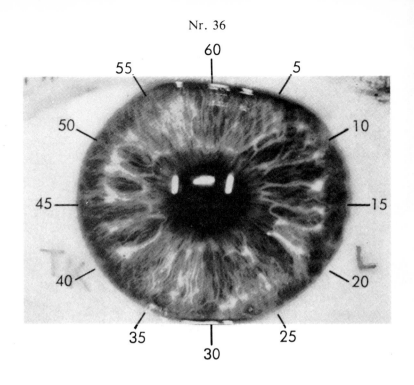

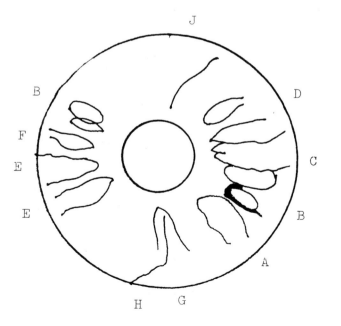

Iris 36—left

Nr. 37

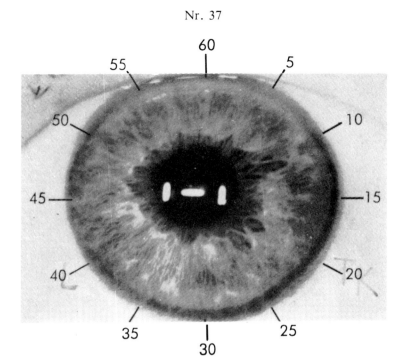

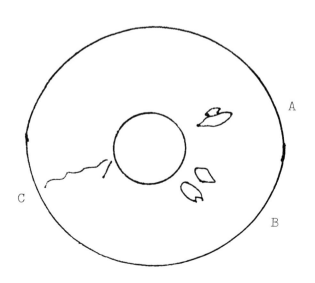

Iris 37—left

Nr. 38

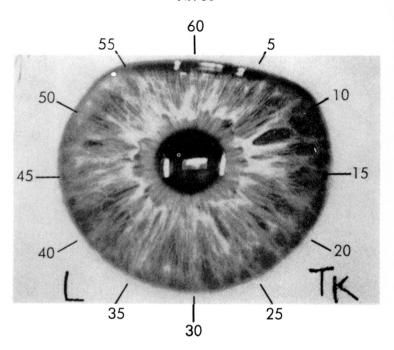

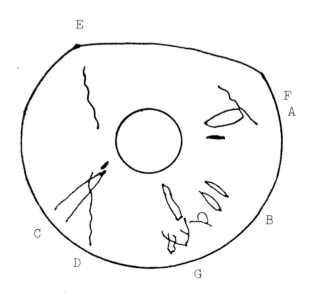

Iris 38—left

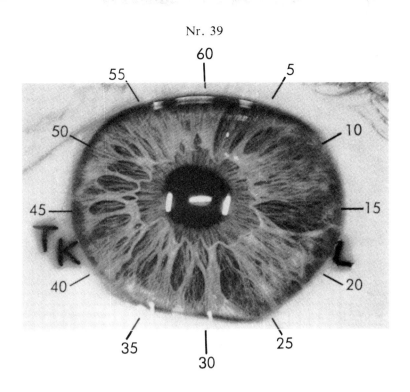

Nr. 39

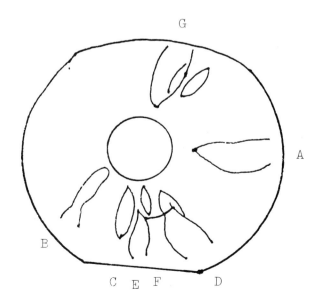

Iris 39—left

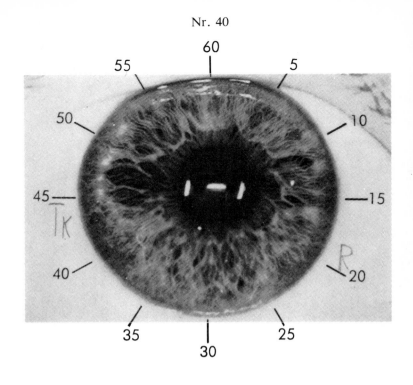

Nr. 40

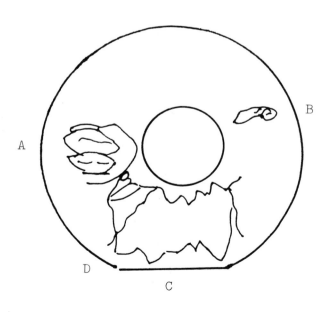

Iris 40—right

Nr. 41

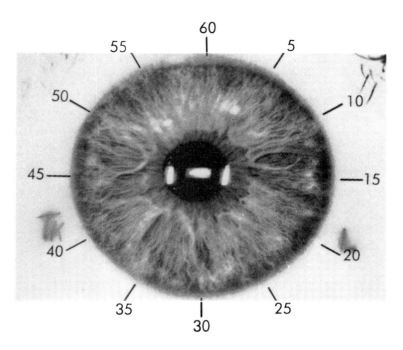

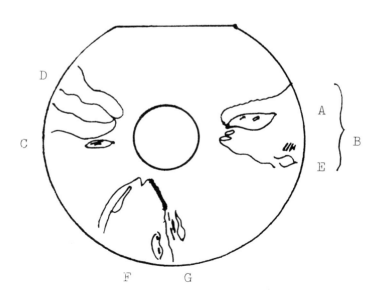

Iris 41—left

Nr. 42

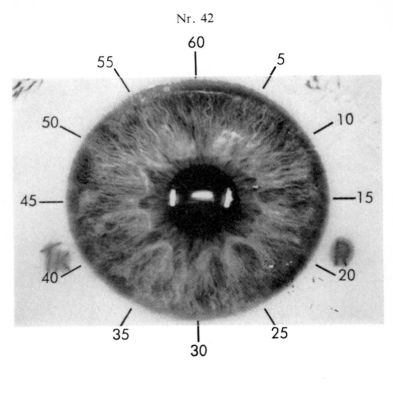

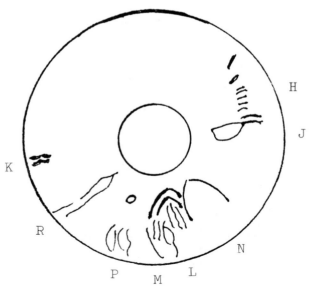

Iris 42—right

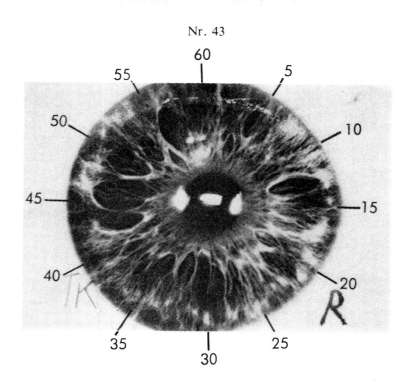

Nr. 43

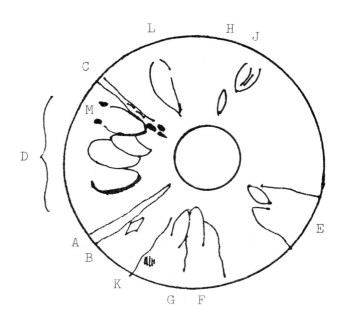

Iris 43—right

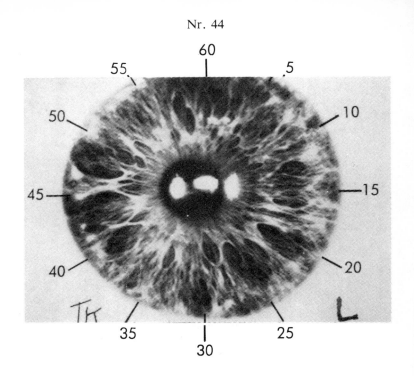

Nr. 44

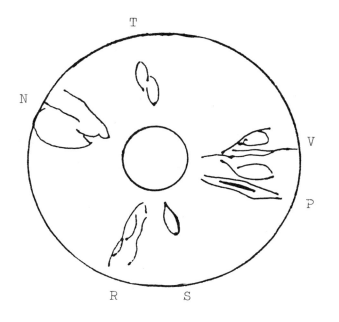

Iris 44—left

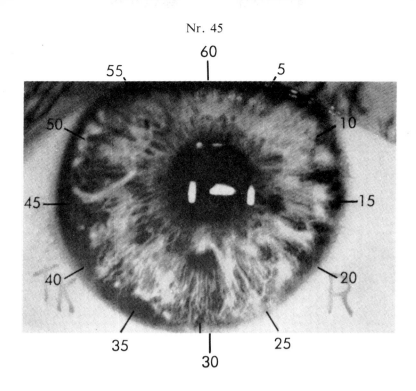

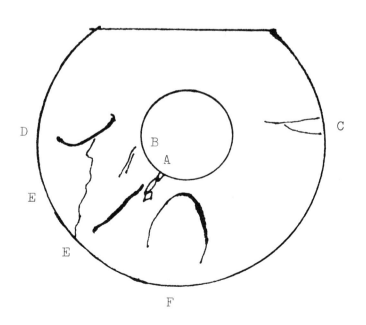

Iris 45—right

Nr. 46

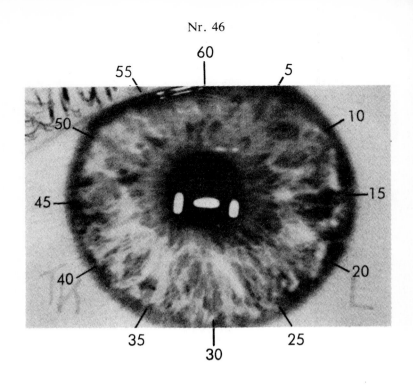

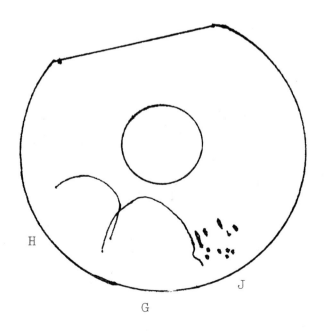

Iris 46—left

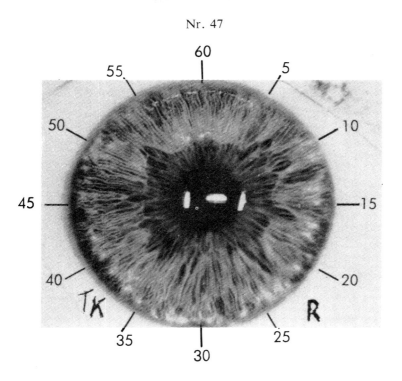

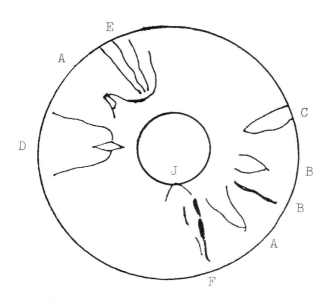

Iris 47—right

Nr. 48

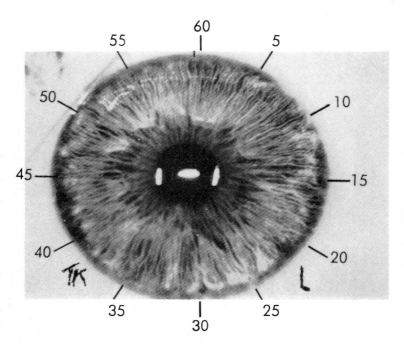

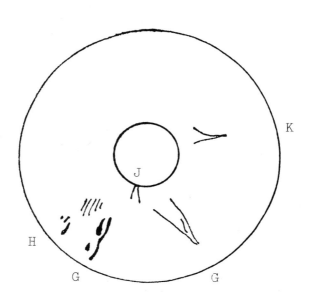

Iris 48—left

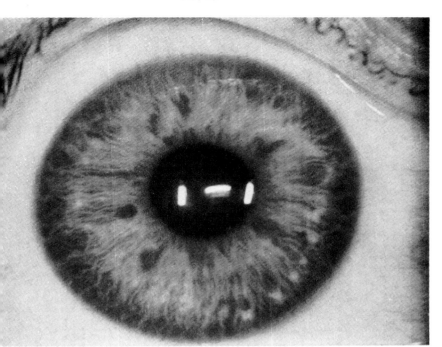

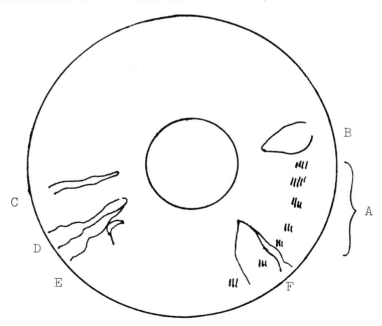

Iris 49—right

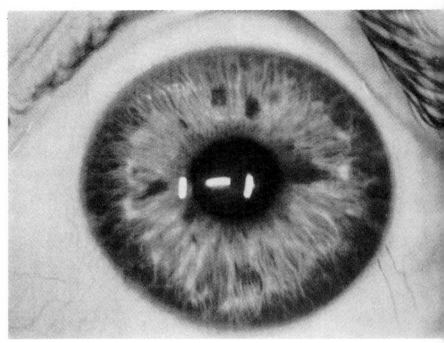

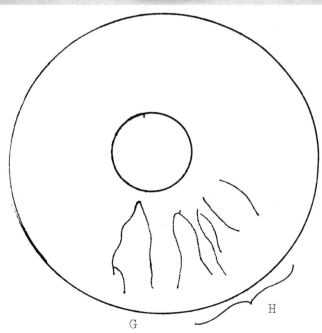

G   H

Iris 50—left

Nr. 51

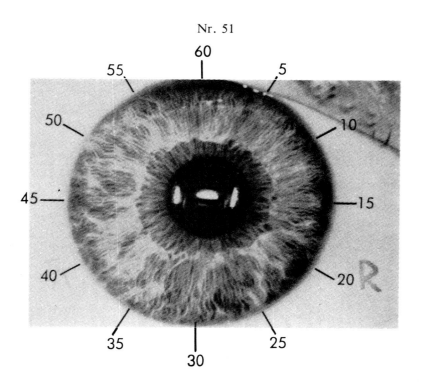

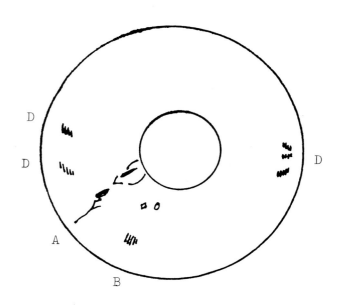

Iris 51—right

Nr. 52

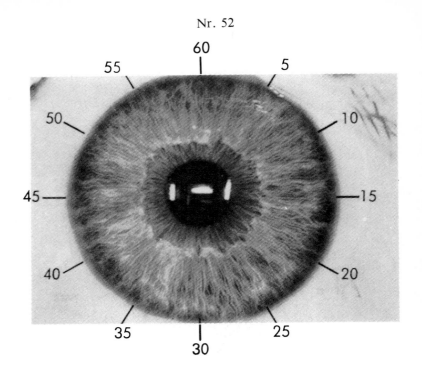

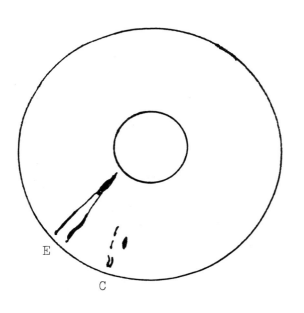

Iris 52—left

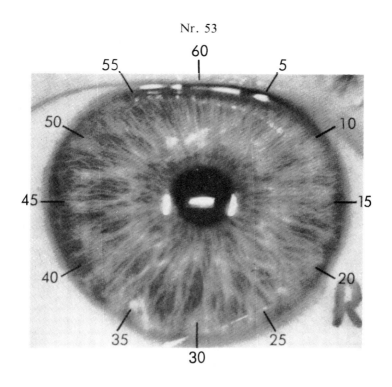

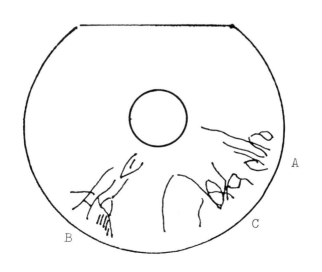

Iris 53—right

Nr. 54

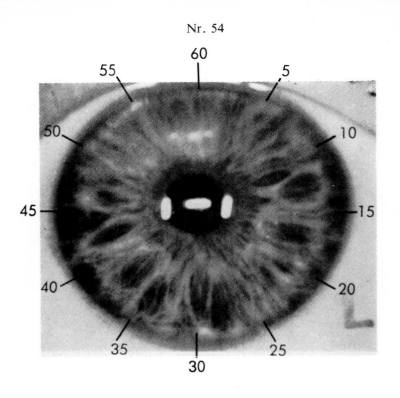

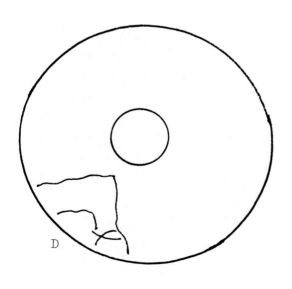

Iris 54—left

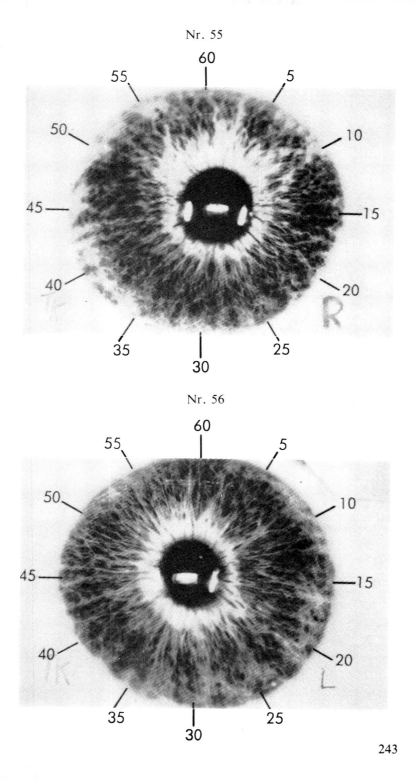

Nr. 55

Nr. 56